BIOCHEMISTRY RESEARCH TRENDS

FORSKOLIN

SOURCES, MECHANISMS OF ACTION AND HEALTH EFFECTS

BIOCHEMISTRY RESEARCH TRENDS

Additional books in this series can be found on Nova's website under the Series tab.

Additional e-books in this series can be found on Nova's website under the e-book tab.

BIOCHEMISTRY RESEARCH TRENDS

FORSKOLIN

SOURCES, MECHANISMS OF ACTION AND HEALTH EFFECTS

MARTY H. WALKER
EDITOR

NOVINKA

New York

Library of Congress Cataloging-in-Publication Data

ISBN: 978-1-63463-918-7
Library of Congress Control Number: 2014960016

Published by Nova Science Publishers, Inc. † New York

CONTENTS

PREFACE

Forskolin is a labdane diterpene, isolated from plant *Coleus forskohlii* (Lamiaceae), which has been used in traditional Indian medicine, Ayurveda. Forskolin increases the production of cyclic adenosine monophosphatase (cAMP) by activating adenylate cyclase. Forskolin has many pharmacological effects and some of them are independent of cAMP. *Coleus forskohlii* root, which contains forskolin has been used in Ayurvedic medicine for cardiovascular disorders and gastrointestinal disorders. Recently, forskolin has been used as anti-obesity and anti-glaucoma agents. This book discusses the sources, mechanisms of action and health effects of forskolin.

Chapter 1 - Sun sensitivity and skin cancer risk are largely determined by skin complexion. Dark skin, which is UV- and cancer-resistant, is characterized by abundant deposition of melanin pigment in the epidermis. Melanin, which acts as a "sunblock" to physically interfere with penetration of damaging UV rays into the skin, is a pigment made by melanocytes that are positioned at the dermal-epidermal junction. Skin complexion is a polymorphic phenotype regulated by a number of genetic loci, however one of the most relevant to melanization of the skin and melanoma risk is the melanocortin 1 receptor (MC1R). Among human populations, loss-of-function of MC1R signaling due to inherited polymorphisms in the MC1R gene, are associated with a fair-skinned undermelanized, UV-sensitive and melanoma-prone phenotype. MC1R signaling, which is mediated by cAMP second messenger generation, can be pharmacologically stimulated by topical application of forskolin, a skin-permeable labdane diterpene which directly activates adenylyl cyclase. Here, the authors review skin physiology, focusing on the MC1R signaling pathway and pharmacologic induction of epidermal melanin and enhanced DNA repair by forskolin.

Chapter 2 - *Purpose:* The aim of the present work was to show the potential neuroprotective activity of forskolin, a receptor-independent activator of adenylate-cyclase, in an experimental model of ocular hypertension in the rat.

Methods: Methylcellulose at 2% was injected into the anterior chamber of rat eyes to induce IOP elevation. Animals were either treated or not with forskolin (1 mg/Kg) in their diet.

Results: Seven days after IOP elevation, rat retinas were evaluated for apoptosis (TUNEL and caspase 3) and iNOS. Forskolin treatment resulted in a reduced increase of IOP after methylcellulose injection, and a decreased production of iNOS, that resulted in a reduced expression of caspase 3 and TUNEL positive cells.

Conclusion: The combined action on IOP and neuron survival suggests a neuroprotective activity of forskolin in glaucomatous neurodegenerative disease, in which elevated IOP is the main risk factor, but not the only determinant of the progressive death of retinal ganglion cells.

Chapter 3 - Since 1971, forskolin has been widely used in research because it activates the ATP pyrophosphate-lyase (cyclizing) enzyme system, EC 4.6.1.1 (adenylate cyclase, AC), resulting in increased cAMP levels. Recently, this terpene has been used as a natural supplement to treat arterial hypertension and asthma through its ability to relax blood vessels. However, animal models have suggested that forskolin may have potential embryotoxicity and teratogenicity in human embryos.

Studies show that forskolin is dangerous to the cardiovascular system in developing chick embryos at Hamburger-Hamilton stage 24 (HH24), a stage in which the developing cardiovascular system is modulated by catecholamines. This chapter studies forskolin-induced morphological changes in the cardiovascular system, even when applied in embryos at the HH12 stage, which is characterized by the absence of the catecholaminergic machinery. Eggs containing chick embryos that were incubated for 48 h (HH12-13) were grouped into basal, control and test groups. Embryos were assayed *in ovo* by injection of 10 µl of forskolin solutions (1.07×10^{-12} mol/egg; 4.14×10^{-12} mol/egg; 8.29×10^{-12} mol/egg; 15.58×10^{-12} mol/egg; 33.16×10^{-12} mol/egg and 66.33×10^{-12} mol/egg) in the air camera of the yolk sac. The basal group did not receive an injection, while the control group was injected with 10 µl of distilled water. No lethality was observed at HH18, when the morphology of the area vasculosa (AV) and the whole embryo was observed. In eggs from the test group, the phenotype of both the AV and the embryo were disrupted depending on the amount of forskolin injected. In contrast, normal cardiovascular development was observed in the AV and in the whole embryos from the basal and control groups.

In conclusion, forskolin is potentially toxic for extraembryonic vascular tissues and embryonic cardiovascular system development, even at stages where this system is resistant to catecholamines. These results suggest that forskolin is contraindicated for women who are planning a pregnancy.

Chapter 4 - Forskolin is a labdane diterpene, isolated from plant *Coleus forskohlii* (Lamiaceae), which has been used in traditional Indian medicine, Ayurveda. Forskolin (7beta-acetoxy-8, 13-epoxy-1a, 6β, 9a-trihydroxy-labd-14-en-11-one) increases the production of cyclic adenosine monophosphatase (cAMP) byactivating adenylate cyclase. Forskolin has many pharmacological effects and some of them are independent of cAMP. *Coleus forskohlii* root, which contains forskolin has been used in Ayurvedic medicine for cardiovascular disorders and gastrointestinal disorders. Recently, forskolin has been used as anti-obesity and anti-glaucoma agents. This chapter aims to summarize pharmacological studies of forskolin towards its clinical applications especially for obesity and metabolic syndrome.

In: Forskolin
Editor: Marty H. Walker
ISBN: 978-1-63463-918-7

Chapter 1

UV PROTECTION OF THE SKIN BY TOPICALLY-APPLIED FORSKOLIN

Alexandra Amaro-Ortiz,[1], Mary Boulanger[2] and John D'Orazio[3,*]
[1]University of Kentucky College of Medicine, Markey Cancer Center and the Graduate Center for Toxicology, Lexington, KY, US
[2]University of Kentucky and the Markey Cancer Center, Lexington, KY, US
[3]University of Kentucky College of Medicine, Markey Cancer Center, The Graduate Center for Toxicology and the Department of Pediatrics, Lexington, KY, US

ABSTRACT

Sun sensitivity and skin cancer risk are largely determined by skin complexion. Dark skin, which is UV- and cancer-resistant, is characterized by abundant deposition of melanin pigment in the epidermis. Melanin, which acts as a "sunblock" to physically interfere with penetration of damaging UV rays into the skin, is a pigment made by melanocytes that are positioned at the dermal-epidermal junction. Skin complexion is a polymorphic phenotype regulated by a number of genetic loci, however one of the most relevant to melanization of the skin and

* Author to whom correspondence should be addressed; e-mail: jdorazio@uky.edu; Tel.: 859-323-6238; Fax: 859-257-8940.

melanoma risk is the melanocortin 1 receptor (MC1R). Among human populations, loss-of-function of MC1R signaling due to inherited polymorphisms in the MC1R gene, are associated with a fair-skinned undermelanized, UV-sensitive and melanoma-prone phenotype. MC1R signaling, which is mediated by cAMP second messenger generation, can be pharmacologically stimulated by topical application of forskolin, a skin-permeable labdane diterpene which directly activates adenylyl cyclase. Here, we review skin physiology, focusing on the MC1R signaling pathway and pharmacologic induction of epidermal melanin and enhanced DNA repair by forskolin.

SKIN

Being the largest organ of the body, the skin accounts for around 16% of total body mass. Fully developed skin consists of epithelial, mesenchymal, glandular, and neurovascular components that together compose the two primary layers of the skin – the epidermis and the dermis. The epidermis is the outermost layer of the skin, derived from ectoderm and charged with physically protecting the body from physical, chemical and microbiologic external threats [1, 2]. The epidermis is primarily made up of keratinocytes, which express cytokeratins and form desmosomes and tight junctions to maintain an effective physicochemical barrier. The epidermis is classified into functional layers by keratinocyte characteristics, including size, shape, nucleation, and keratin expression (Figure 1) [3]. The epidermis is a self-renewing tissue, characterized by the constant division of keratinocyte stem cells in the basal layer to form nascent epidermal keratinocytes. As these cells are pushed outward by further proliferation of keratinocyte stem cells, they differentiate as they migrate to the surface of the skin, accumulating keratin, pigment and forming tight junctions with each other. Ultimately keratinocytes form corneocytes which are dead yet intact cells that create the protective barrier of the epidermis through tight-linkages [4-7]. The dermis, positioned directly beneath the epidermis, can be thought of as a supportive layer with most dermal cells being derived from mesoderm. The dermis contains a variety of important cutaneous structures, including hair follicles, nerves, blood vessels and sebaceous glands and sweat glands. Immune cells and fibroblasts are also housed in dermis and participate in immune responses and extracellular matrix and collagen formation, respectively. The dermis and epidermis are separated by a very thin basement membrane.

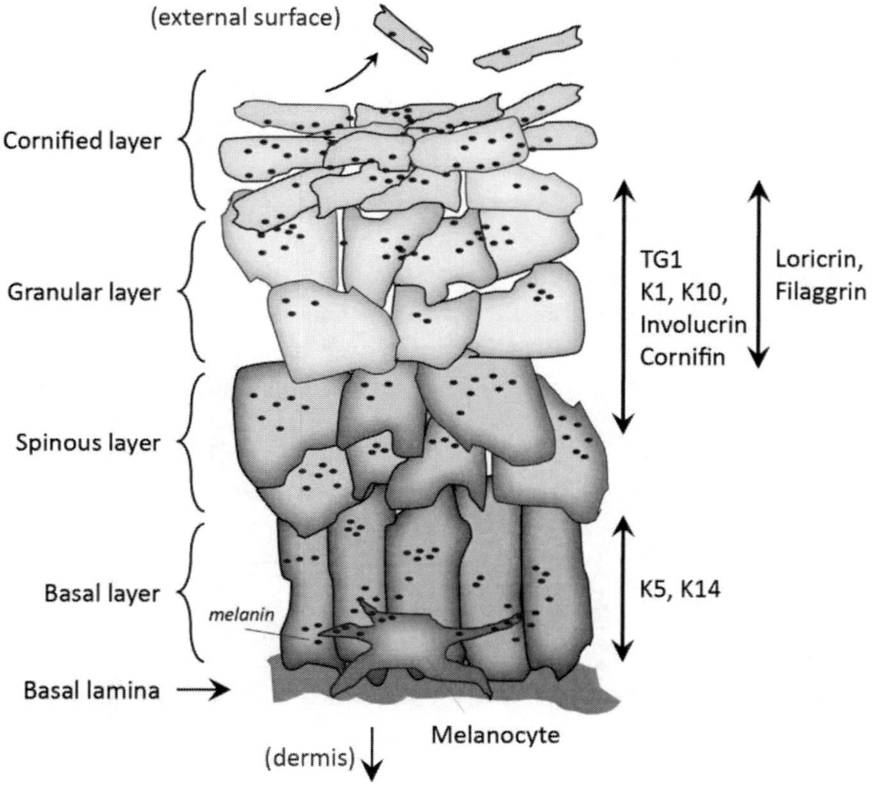

Figure 1. Structure of the epidermis. Predominantly made up of keratinocytes derived from stem cells in the basal layer, the epidermis is a self-renewing tissue in which keratinocytes undergo a programmed series of differentiating events (e.g. formation of tight junctions, accumulation of cytokeratin, cornification, loss of nuclei) as they make their way to the skin's surface. Along the way, they accumulate melanin produced by melanocytes to provide physical protection against UV radiation. Epidermal layers are generally defined by keratinocyte morphology and expression of cytokeratins and other proteins. Largely because of its physico-chemical properties, the epidermis provides a critical barrier against microbial, chemical and toxic agents such as UV.

Keratinocytes protect the skin from UV penetration by accumulating melanin pigments during their maturation. The skin is organized functionally into "epidermal melanin units" wherein many keratinocytes interact with one melanocyte. Melanin pigment, most of which is found in keratinocytes in the skin, is actually manufactured in melanocytes, the second most common cell type in the epidermis [8]. Each melanocyte transfers melanin pigments to interdigitating keratinocytes in its particular epidermal melanin unit. In this way, pigment is produced in epidermal melanocytes (typically found just above the basement membrane in the basal layer) and accumulates in keratinocytes. Melanin in keratinocytes effectively blocks penetration of UV radiation into the skin and is therefore a critical mediator of UV protection [9].

SKIN CANCER AND MELANOMA

Taken together and including both keratinocyte and melanocyte malignancies, skin cancers are by far the most numerous cancers diagnosed today. Fortunately, most are keratinocyte-derived basal cell or squamous cell carcinomas, which are effectively treated surgically and generally have good outcomes.

Table 1. Major melanoma risk factors

Age	**The incidence of melanoma increases dramatically with age.**
• Sun exposure	Occupational or recreational UV exposure, living in UV-rich geographies (e.g. equatorial locations), living at altitude.
• Tanning bed use	First exposure to indoor tanning before 35 years of age raises lifetime risk of melanoma by 75%
• Fair Skin Complexion	Deficiency of the highly UV-protective eumelanin epidermal pigment allows more UV to penetrate into the skin and promote mutagenesis.
• Chronic exposure to heavy metals	Chromium, cobalt and other metals may promote oxidative mutagenesis in melanocytes.
• Poor ability to tan	A propensity to burn rather than tan after sun exposure correlates with increased melanoma risk.
• History of sunburn	One or more severe blistering sunburns as a child or teenager increases risk
• Personal history of melanoma	Once a person has been diagnosed with a melanoma, their risk for others is heightened. Up to 10% of melanoma patients will develop a second melanoma in their lifetime.
• Family history of melanoma	Inherited CDKN2A defects (the gene that encodes the p16INK4A and p14ARFtumor suppressors) is associated with familial melanoma
• Having a large number of moles (nevi)	Many melanomas appear to arise from pre-existing moles. Benign nevi and melanoma both frequently exhibit gain-of-function mutation in the B-Raf gene.
• Immune suppression	Immunosuppressive therapies, for example, as used to prevent rejection of solid organs in transplant recipients, is associated with melanoma.
• DNA repair deficiency	Xeroderma pigmentosum (XP) patients who lack one of at least eight enzymes in a common nucleotide excision repair (NER) pathway have a 2,000-fold increased risk of skin cancers, including melanoma.

Melanoma, on the other hand, accounts for almost 10,000 deaths each year in the US alone, despite representing a small fraction of the total number of skin malignancies [10]. Melanoma derives from melanocytes, is generally resistant to treatment and is prone to spreading throughout the body from is site of origin (usually in the epidermis). For a variety of reasons, the prevalence of melanoma has been steadily increasing in Western countries for decades. Whereas only one in approximately 1,500 Americans was diagnosed with melanoma in his/her lifetime in the 1930's, today that number has increased to roughly one in sixty people. Many risk factors for melanoma have been identified (Table 1) [11-17].

UV exposure is thought to be a causal factor in the majority of melanoma cases. UV exposure in the form of sunlight or purposeful artificial tanning, is determined by many factors including occupational and recreational outdoor activities, indoor tanning, amount of clothing/sun protection worn as well as proximity to the equator and altitude. Tanning bed use in particular has garnered much attention as a potentially important melanoma contributing factor. Meta-analytic studies have estimated that indoor tanning bed use before the age of thirty five, for example, increases lifetime risk of melanoma by as much as 75% [12]. Clearly the more UV a person is exposed to (particularly strong intermittent doses such as those that cause sunburns), the higher his/her risk of melanoma.

MELANIN

A key determinant for UV sensitivity and skin cancer risk is skin complexion, which is determined primarily by the amount and type of melanin present in the epidermis. Melanin is a large bio-aggregate of pigmented chemical species derived from the amino acid tyrosine (Figure 2). Tyrosinase is the rate-limiting biosynthetic enzyme in the melanogenesis pathway, as it catalyzes the first two steps of melanin synthesis (conversion of tyrosine to DOPA and then to DOPAquinone). There are two major "mature" forms of melanin known as eumelanin and pheomelanin. Eumelanin is brown or black pigment and protects against UV exposure by absorbing the energy of photons in the UV spectra, thereby interfering with UV entry into the deep, sensitive layers of the skin. In contrast, pheomelanin is a sulfur-containing pigment that is lighter in color and less able to block UV. In fact, pheomelanin may actually potentiate UV injury to the skin by contributing to free radical formation and oxidative cellular damage. Therefore, individuals with high levels of pheomelanin and low levels of eumelanin in the skin are UV sensitive and are at a greater risk for developing skin cancers including melanoma [18, 19].

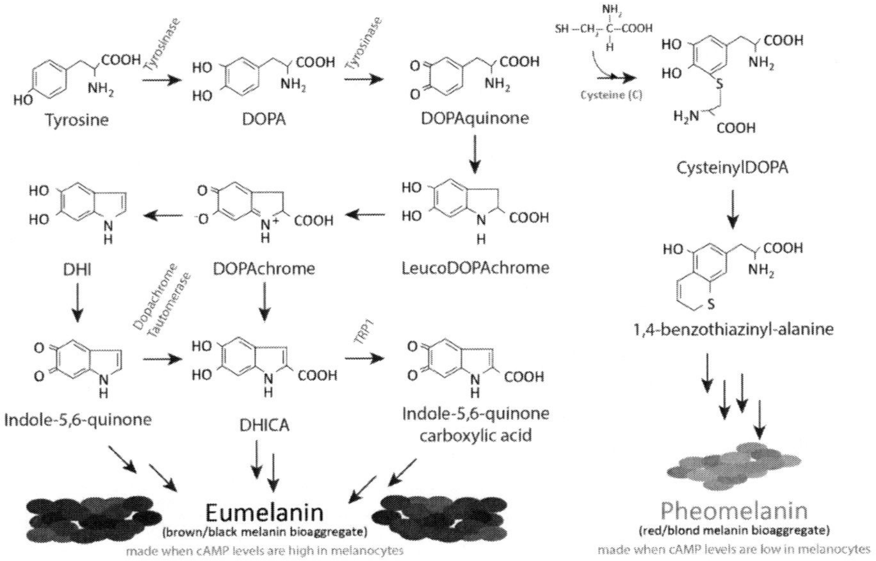

Figure 2. Melanin synthesis. Melanin is a large bio-aggregate made up of pigmented chemical species derived from the amino acid tyrosine. Tyrosinase is the enzyme that catalyzes the first two stages of melanin biosynthesis. Albinism, caused by an inability to synthesize melanin pigments, results from tyrosinase deficiency. There are two major forms of melanin: (1) eumelanin, a brown/black species quite effective at blocking UV photons, and (2) pheomelanin, a red/blonde sulfur-containing UV-permeable pigment. Epidermal melanin content is a mixture of eumelanin and pheomelanin, with skin complexion being mainly determined by eumelanin levels.

Melanocytes generally manufacture both types of melanin, however the ratio of eumelanin-to-pheomelanin and the total amount of melanin made vary depending on a variety of inherited and environmental factors. In general, eumelanin production is favored when cytoplasmic cAMP levels are high, whereas pheomelanin is synthesized when melanocytic cAMP levels are low. As will be expounded on below, proper signaling through the MSH-MC1R hormonal axis (which signals melanocytes through cAMP second messenger generation) is a major regulator of eumelanin synthesis and accumulation in the skin [20-22].

SKIN PIGMENTATION

Skin complexion is a complex phenotype, regulated both by inherited and environmental factors. Several genes control basal melanin type and melanin levels of the skin [23]. Much is known about pigment determinants through the study of mouse coat color mutants such as *extension*, slaty or pink-eyed dilution [24]. Many of the genes regulating epidermal melanization are localized to melanosomes, the intracellular organelles in which melanin biosynthesis occurs in melanocytes. Many, like tyrosinase, are directly involved in melanin synthesis. Tyrosinase deficiency, with abundant examples throughout the animal kingdom, is associated with oculocutaneous albinism in which melanocytes make neither eumelanin nor pheomelanin in adequate amount and affected individuals display an albino phenotype. Not surprisingly, such persons are highly UV-sensitive and tend to avoid outdoor activities that risk significant exposure to ambient sunlight. Defects in other pigment biosynthesis loci tend to have a less stark phenotype, typically causing melanin dilution phenotypes rather than absolute albinism as tyrosinase loss does. Other pigment-determining genes are involved in melanocyte migration and/or differentiation and result in loss of melanocytes in discreet anatomic compartments. Microphthalmia (Mitf), for example, is a master melanocytic differentiation factor and is necessary for melanocyte development. Mitf mutations are associated with the absence of melanocytes in the skin and other tissues. One particular type of Waardenburg syndrome, associated with Mitf-related absence of melanocytes in the inner ear for example, is exemplified by hearing loss. Similarly, Kit ligand regulates melanocyte migration and defects in Kit ligand are associated with segmental melanocyte absence (piebaldism). Certain genes regulate either the ratio or absolute levels of eumelanin or pheomelanin produced by melanocytes. Solute carrier family 24 member 5 (SLC24A5), whose product is thought to be a melanosomal cation exchange protein, may account for up to 40% of skin color differences between Europeans and Africans [25]. Clearly several genetic loci determine human skin complexion through regulation of the amount and type of melanin in the epidermis.

Human skin pigmentation can be described according to the Fitzpatrick Scale, which classifies human skin tone based on basal pigmentation (Figure 3). Cutaneous response to UV and skin cancer risk can largely be predicted by skin complexion and melanin levels. The lowest amount of UV required to cause a sunburn, called the minimal erythematous dose (MED), is one indication of UV sensitivity. Fair-skinned persons with little UV-blocking eumelanin in the skin are much more likely to get a sunburn after UV exposure, and therefore have much lower MED's than their heavily melanized counterparts who are well protected from UV. UV sensitivity also informs skin cancer risk, including melanoma.

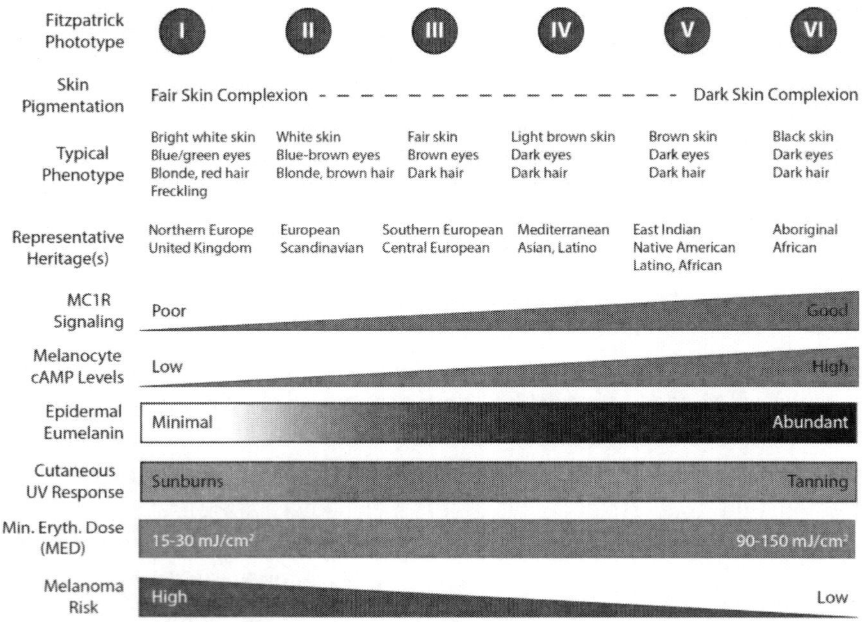

Figure 3. Human skin complexion, melanocyte physiology and melanoma risk. Skin complexion, described by "Fitzpatrick Scale" ranging from very fair (type I) to very dark (type VI), is determined largely by eumelanin content in the epidermis. Though many genes control melanization of the skin, the MC1R is a critical mediator of adaptive pigmentation (tanning) and melanoma risk. Fair-skinned individuals with low levels of melanin in the epidermis display a UV sensitive phenotype, tending to burn rather than tan, after UV exposure. Individuals harboring loss-of-function MC1R polymorphisms tend to have undermelanized skin that permits UV entry, predisposing them to melanoma and other skin cancer. Such individuals may also accumulate more mutations from UV because of defective DNA repair. Minimal erythematous dose (MED) is defined as the least amount of UV that causes inflammation of the skin 24–48 h after exposure (i.e., the lowest UV dose that causes sunburn).

Being of low Fitzpatrick phototype, for example, correlates not only with tendency to burn rather than tan but also with higher lifetime incidence of melanoma and other skin cancers.

Melanocortin 1 Receptor (MC1R)

One of the most important pigment-regulating genes is the melanocortin 1 receptor (MC1R), located on chromosome 16q24.3 in the human. The MC1R protein product, made up of 317 amino acids and having a molecular mass of

34.7 kDa, is localized to the external membrane of melanocytes. It is a transmembrane protein that spans the plasma membrane 7 times and is a G_s-coupled hormonal receptor (Figure 4).

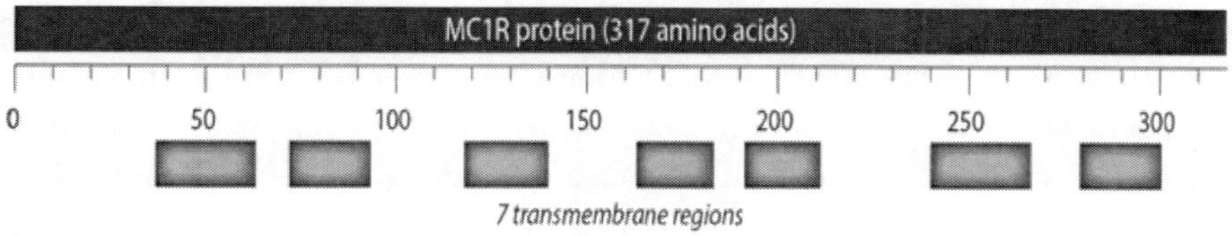

Figure 4. MC1R protein structure. The human melanocortin 1 receptor (MC1R) is made up of 317 amino acids, and contains 7 transmembrane domains which facilitate its orientation in the plasma membrane.

In the mouse, loss of MC1R on the C57BL/6J background is sufficient to essentially "flip" pigment phenotype from a jet black, heavily melanized condition to a blonde/red fair complexion. Thus, the MC1R is a major regulator of melanin biosynthesis, controlling the ratio of eumelanin to pheomelanin produced in the skin and hair of many species [26, 27]. Pheomelanotic, UV-sensitive phenotypes based on MC1R dysfunction are evident in a variety of mammals, including humans. MC1R dysfunction may have been evolutionarily selected in human populations that migrated away from equatorial, warm and UV-rich climates in order to reduce risk of vitamin D deficiency in environments wherein UV is less abundant. A heavily melanized epidermis in such climates might predispose to rickets, a debilitating metabolic disorder of calcium imbalance and bone demineralization due to inadequate UV-induced vitamin D production. Thus, loss of function polymorphisms of MC1R are common in people of Northern European descent, and millions of people harbor MC1R polymorphisms that interfere with melanization of the skin. Three major human MC1R polymorphisms – Arg151Cys (R151C), Arg160Trp (R160W) and Asp294His (D294H) – are collectively known as "red hair color" (RHC) mutations because they correlate with basal red/blonde hair coloration [22]. Importantly, MC1R loss of function polymorphisms also correlate with a very UV-sensitive and skin cancer-prone phenotype. Thus although MC1R mutations may reduce risk for vitamin D deficiency, such persons have up to a four-fold increased lifetime risk for melanoma [28].

Functional MC1R deficiency contributes to carcinogenesis of melanocytes in a variety of ways, all of which are relevant to melanocyte UV physiologic responses. First, because MC1R function is needed for adaptive pigmentation (i.e. tanning), persons lacking robust MC1R signaling have a blunted melanin response to UV. Having a fairer skin complexion allows more UV radiation to enter the skin, leading to a larger mutagenic burden than if the skin were protected by more eumelanin. Second, MC1R signaling directly influences melanocytes' ability to repair and cope with cellular UV damage. We and others have shown that MC1R-intact melanocytes clear UV photolesions faster and better than those without adequate MC1R function [28-33]. This implies that MC1R-defective persons suffer more UV penetration into the epidermis and that melanocytes can't repair UV damage adequately and are therefore at higher risk of malignant degeneration. Third, emerging evidence suggests an important anti-oxidant role for MC1R, implying that MC1R protects melanocytes against UV-mediated free radical injury. Oxidative UV damage is clearly mutagenic and may be an important contributor to melanoma development [30, 34-36]. Lastly, Mitra and colleagues showed that MC1R dysfunction leads to melanocyte damage and melanoma formation even in the absence of UV through oxidative damage caused by pheomelanin expression [37]. Taken together, abundant evidence exists to position MC1R as a critical mediator of melanocyte cancer resistance.

The MSH-MC1R Hormonal Axis

As a G_s-coupled protein receptor, MC1R signals its activation by recruiting adenylyl cyclase to convert ATP into the second messenger cAMP [38]. Elevation of melanocyte cAMP levels leads to pro-differentiation and pro-survival changes in melanocytes, including melanin synthesis and UV resistance. Importantly, cAMP-mediated UV protection appears to occur regardless of whether it is induced through receptor (MC1R) stimulation or pharmacologically by adenylyl cyclase activation or phosphodiesterase inhibition [39-44]. When cAMP levels are high, melanocytes are stimulated to produce eumelanin. When cAMP levels are low, pheomelanin is made instead by default. As mentioned above, cAMP also increases melanocyte survival after UV, enhances DNA repair and genome maintenance pathways and induces various anti-oxidant cellular defenses. Altogether, cAMP promotes a wide variety of melanocyte protective responses.

MC1R signaling and its downstream effector responses are heavily influenced by soluble ligands. Alpha melanocyte stimulating hormone (α-MSH) is a melanocortin and among the most important MC1R ligands present in the skin. α-MSH is produced as a cleavage product of the pro-opiomelanocortin (POMC) peptide [45], itself induced in a damage-dependent manner in epidermal keratinocytes after exposure to UV [46]. α-MSH is a 13 amino acid oligopeptide (Ac-SYSMEHFRWGKPV-NH_2) with potent agonistic activity at the MC1R. α-MSH-MC1R interactions promote melanocyte adenylyl cyclase activation and up-regulation of cAMP production and all of the downstream UV protective responses. MC1R signaling can also be influenced by "weaker" melanocortins, including β-MSH, γ-MSH and adrenocorticotropic hormone (ACTH). Thus, melanocyte cAMP levels are regulated not only by MC1R structure (i.e. presence of polymorphisms) but also by the amount of melanocortins expressed in the skin [26, 47].

Intriguingly, there are at least two non-melanocortin proteins present in the skin that oppose α-MSH effects to down-regulate MC1R signaling: agouti signaling protein (ASIP) and beta-defensin 3 (BD3). Although little is known about ASIP and BD3 function in UV responses, these MC1R antagonists may serve important regulatory functions (e.g. shutting down or limiting the MC1R signaling cascade in the skin). ASIP binds to MC1R with high affinity to blocks α-MSH effect and potently down-regulate melanocyte cAMP levels [39, 48]. BD3, long known to be an important innate antimicrobial peptide produced in the skin, seems to be able to blunt both α-MSH and ASIP signaling effects at the MC1R [49, 50]. Thus, regulation of MC1R signaling in the context of whole skin is likely to be complex and multifactorial. Nonetheless, the physiologic and molecular events that mediate adaptive pigmentation (tanning) after UV radiation serve to illustrate central concepts of the MSH-MC1R signaling axis (Figure 5).

K14-Scf Transgenic Model of the Fair-Skinned Human

The use of mice as an animal model to investigate pigment-dependent physiology in the skin is limited because of innate differences between human skin and mouse skin. Whereas human skin maintains melanocytes in the epidermis throughout life to impart melanin pigments to the epidermis, mouse skin is only transiently populated by melanocytes in the epidermis in the neonatal period. After the first few days of life, mouse skin lacks epidermal melanocytes as they only transiently migrate through on their way to the dermal hair follicles, and there is no significant pigmentation of actual epidermal skin in contrast to the fur which is heavily pigmented because of localization and retention of follicular melanocytes. In humans, a population of melanocytes in remains localized to the basal layer, maintained there because of the production of KIT ligand (also known as stem cell factor, or SCF) from basal keratinocytes [51, 52]. cKIT signaling promotes melanocyte survival and differentiation [53]. For unknown reasons, there is little SCF expression in the epidermis of mice beyond the neonatal period and as a result, melanocytes are not retained in epidermis except for minor populations in the ears, tails and footpads. Thus, even though striking pigment differences may exist in coat color between strains, the skin between hairs in most of the skin remains unpigmented (pink).

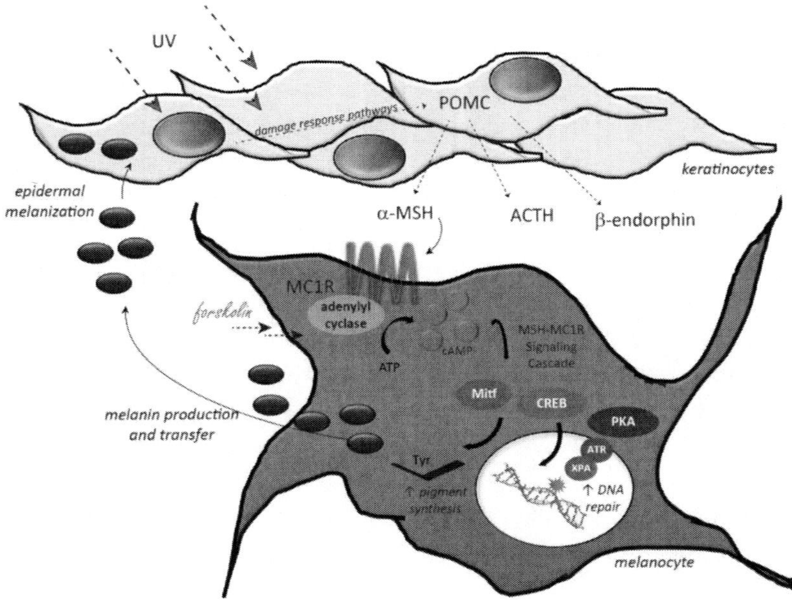

Figure 5. The MSH-MC1R signaling cascade and adaptive melanization. When UV radiation strikes the skin, keratinocytes in the epidermis sustain cellular injury. Canonical DNA and cellular damage response pathways (e.g. p53 activation) are activated, resulting in transcriptional up-regulation of the pro-opiomelanocortin (POMC) gene. The POMC propeptide is processed and cleaved into several proteolytic components, including alpha melanocyte stimulating hormone (α-MSH), adrenocorticotropic hormone (ACTH) and β-endorphin, a natural opioid. In this way, epidermal α-MSH production is increased, and its secretion from keratinocytes results in paracrine activity with melanocortin 1 receptors (MC1R) on interdigitating melanocytes in the epidermis. MSH-MC1R interactions induce activation of adenylyl cyclase and robust generation of the second messenger cAMP. Elevation of melanocytic cAMP triggers a number of downstream events including activation of protein kinase A and up-regulation of both the cAMP responsive binding element (CREB) and microphthalmia (Mitf) transcription factors. Melanin production is favored by induction of tyrosinase and other melanin biosynthetic enzymes and eumelanin pigments are synthesized and exported to epidermal keratinocytes where they accumulate to protect the skin against further UV exposure. Melanocytic cAMP signaling also enhances genome stability and reduces UV mutagenesis by stimulating nucleotide excision repair (NER) in melanocytes. Thus, the MSH-MC1R-cAMP signaling cascade is UV-protective and reduces risk of malignant degeneration.

One approach to be able to utilize mice to study pigment effects such as forskolin rescue of melanization is to transgenically express melanocyte growth factors such as SCF in the epidermis constitutively throughout life. We initially reported adapting the *K14-Scf* transgenic C57BL/6 mouse model [51] to study melanin effects in the skin [41]. In this model, SCF is constitutively expressed under the control of the human keratin 14 promoter, which is active only in basal keratinocytes. As a result, there is high SCF concentration in the basal layer of the epidermis and melanocytes remain there in abundance throughout life. We showed that melanin expression in the skin was determined by Mc1r signaling status and that it mimicked coat color of the animals [41]. Thus, wild-type $Mc1r^{E/E}$ mice have a jet black appearance of the skin and fur due to robust production of eumelanin.

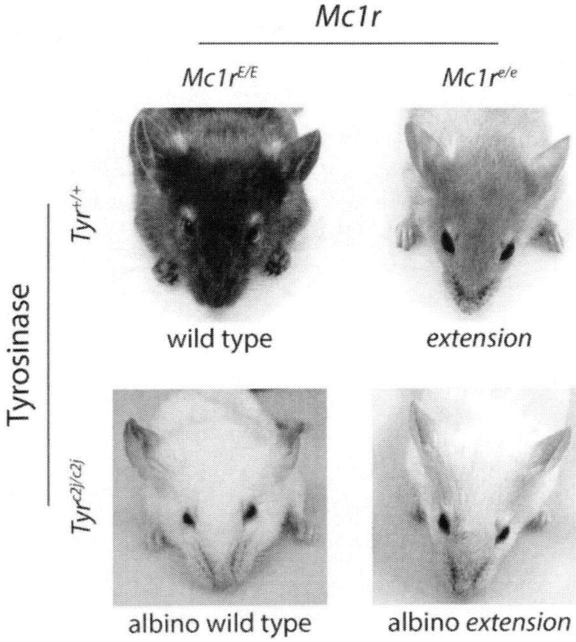

Figure 6. K14-Scf transgenic mouse model. Pigment phenotypes of mice that model human skin of variant melanin and Mc1r composition. Due to the constitutive secretion of stem cell factor (kit ligand) by epidermal keratinocytes, melanocytes are retained in these mice. If tyrosinase is intact, the skin and hair is richly endowed with either eumelanin (when Mc1r is functional) or pheomelanin (when Mc1r is mutated). When tyrosinase is mutant, neither melanin species is expressed, allowing pigment-independent Mc1r effects to be studied. Together, these animals provide a genetically defined system in which to compare melanin and Mc1r influences on cutaneous physiology.

Strikingly, however, animals with mutant Mc1r (known as *extension* mice, or *Mc1r*$^{e/e}$), have fair complexions of the skin and fur due to preferential production of pheomelanin instead. By removing tyrosinase from the system (by incorporating the *c2j* tyrosinase mutation), the animal model can be adapted to isolate Mc1r-pigment independent effects, as neither *Mc1r*$^{E/E}$ "albino wt" nor *Mc1r*$^{e/e}$ "albino *extension*" mice can produce substantial levels of either eumelanin or pheomelanin due to tyrosinase deficiency (Figure 6).

FORSKOLIN

Forskolin, identified in 1974, is a bioactive constituent of the *Coleus forskohlii* (*Plectrantus barbatus*) plant, a perennial herb that grows naturally in subtropical India and Southeast Asia [54]. It was characterized by scientists because the plant from which it was derived had long been used in traditional Ayurvedic medicine for a range of ailments and diseases. The compound, whose chemical name is 17-β-acetoxy-8, 13-epoxy-1α, 6-β, 9α-trihydroxylabd-14-en-11-one, is a direct and rapid activator of adenylyl cyclase. Forskolin's unique heterocyclic structure classifies the molecule as part of the labdane diterpene family (Figure 7).

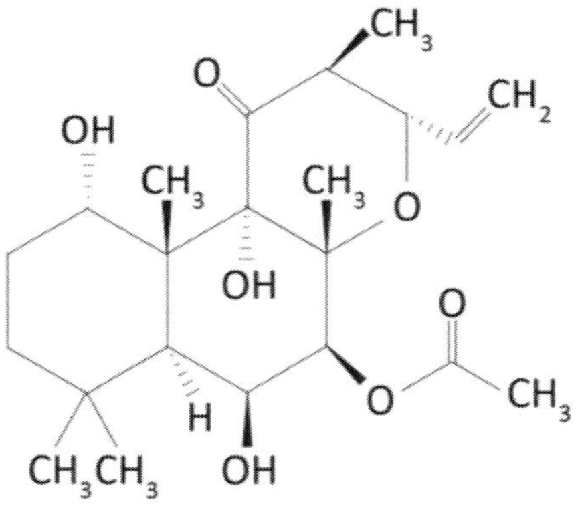

Figure 7. The chemical structure of forskolin, a skin-permeable labdane diterpene.

Forskolin has been reported to be of therapeutic benefit for a variety of different medical conditions including psoriasis, eczema, obesity, menstrual cramping, urinary tract infections and hypertension [55-58], however its lack of selectivity and potential for toxicity (headache, tachycardia) has limited its use [59, 60].

At the molecular level, forskolin binds to adenylyl cyclase, an enzyme that catalyzes production of the second messenger cAMP from ATP. There are nine isoforms of adenylyl cyclase, each regulated by binding of G-protein subunits to control enzymatic activity. Forskolin can bind to all adenylyl cyclase isoforms except adenylyl cyclase 9 [61]. Once activated, adenylyl cyclase changes its conformation to allow the binding of ATP. ATP is then enzymatically converted to cAMP which functions as a potent second messenger involved in signal transduction for a number of intracellular signaling pathways. Because of its hydrophobic nature, forskolin is easily absorbed by the skin and is efficiently absorbed transdermally [62].

Forskolin-Mediated Melanin Rescue

Phenotypic characterization of *Mc1r*-intact vs. –defective mice (heavily pigmented vs. lightly pigmented respectively) offered genetic proof of the importance of Mc1r signaling to melanin production by melanocytes. We reasoned that since Mc1r signals through adenylyl cyclase activation and production of cAMP, that effective melanin production would be cAMP dependent. Indeed, others had reported that the $Mc1r^{e/e}$ *extension* mutation had markedly reduced signaling ability, associated with low levels of cAMP. We reasoned that topical administration of forskolin might effectively increase melanocyte cAMP levels and therefore induce production of eumelanin through its ability to pharmacologically activate adenylyl cyclase.

Using the *K14-Scf* transgenic mouse model, we demonstrated robust induction of eumelanin accumulation in the skin in of $Mc1r^{e/e}$ *extension* (fair-skinned) mice when forskolin was topically applied daily or twice daily for several days (Figure 8) [41, 44]. We found that forskolin stimulated epidermal melanocytes to make and transfer eumelanin to epidermal keratinocytes, mimicking the natural deposition of melanin found in $Mc1r^{E/E}$ wild type mice. We found that forskolin-induced skin pigmentation was dose-dependent and persisted as long as the skin was treated with the drug at least through three months of daily topical applications. Critically, we determined that forskolin-induced epidermal melanin protected against UV exposure, as measured either by interference with UV-induced carcinogenesis [41] or by protection against UV-induced inflammatory changes [42, 44, 63].

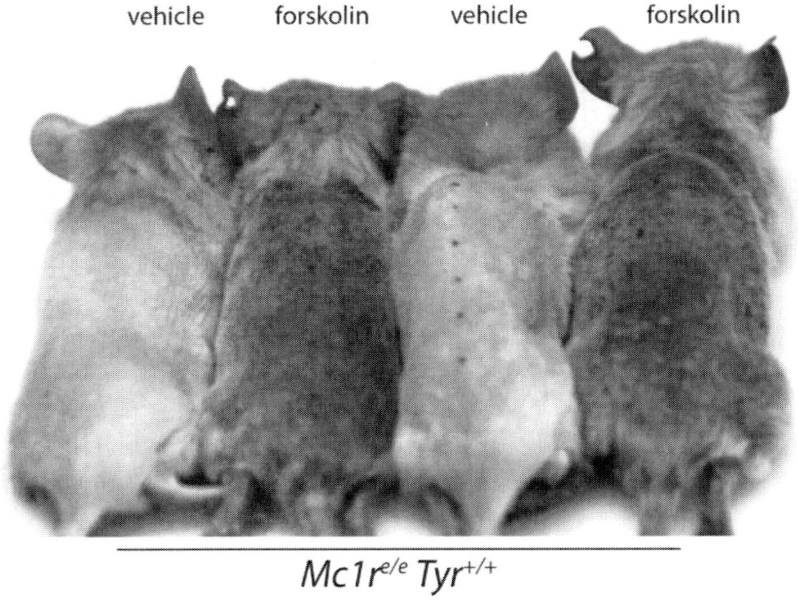

Figure 8. Forskolin-induced melanization of the skin. Pharmacologic induction of epidermal melanin by topically-applied forskolin. *K14-Scf* transgenic *extension* mice (*Mc1r*$^{e/e}$ *Tyr*$^{+/+}$) were treated twice daily with either vehicle (70% ethanol, 30% propylene glycol) or forskolin (prepared as a 20% (w/v) crude root extract). Shown are side-by-side photos of the mice after 14 days. Note the darker skin color of the forskolin-treated mice due to the abundant deposition of eumelanin in the epidermis.

Our prior studies confirmed significant UV protection after 10-15 topical applications of forskolin as measured by "minimal erythematous dose" (MED), the least amount of UV to cause "sun burning" of the skin. In *K14-Scf* transgenic mice, daily topical administration of forskolin promoted epidermal melanization without overt toxicity. After weeks of daily applications, the mice showed no changes in body weight or activity level [42]. Topical forskolin did promote subtle increases in epidermal thickening caused by slight increases in keratinocyte proliferation and thought to be mediated by forskolin-induced keratinocyte growth factor (KGF) expression from fibroblasts in the dermis. Nonetheless, the degree of epidermal thickening was minimal, seemed to reach an equilibrium after approximately 2 weeks of treatment, and was not associated with premalignant or discreet proliferative lesions such as actinic keratosis [42]. Thus we concluded that topically-applied forskolin can pharmacologically "bypass" defective Mc1r signaling and alter the UV-sensitive fair complexion phenotype associated with it. Clearly much more work remains to be done before the full safety and efficacy profile of topical forskolin therapy is understood.

NON-PIGMENT MC1R-MEDIATED UV PROTECTION

Without effective cAMP induction, the skin of MC1R-defective individuals cannot accumulate significant amounts of melanin and therefore is prone to UV damage and carcinogenesis because UV can easily penetrate into the skin. However, the influence of MC1R signaling extends beyond melanization. MC1R signaling facilitates the repair of molecular UV damage in melanocytes, suggesting that MC1R defective persons may be at risk for melanoma not just because they tend to express less melanin in the skin but also because their melanocytes cannot repair DNA damage efficiently [29, 32, 33]. More UV damage coupled with a reduced capacity to reverse UV DNA damage would be predicted to be associated with higher UV mutation rates in melanocytes. Since UV mutations are among the main causative molecular drivers of melanoma, ineffective MC1R signaling directly influences melanoma risk.

NUCLEOTIDE EXCISION REPAIR (NER)

Nucleotide excision repair (NER) is the way in which cells recognize and repair DNA-distorting lesions such as UV-induced DNA damage [64-66]. UV radiation causes specific damage to nucleotides in DNA, particularly among adjacent pyrimidines such as thymidine and cytosine [65]. Through direct absorption of UV energy, the C5-C6 double bond breaks open between neighboring pyrimidines, and new covalent base structures are formed. There are two main UV photolesions. Cyclobutane pyrimidine dimers form when a new 4-member cyclobutyl ring is formed as a result of the C5/C6 bond breakage. Alternatively, a [6-4]-photoproduct is formed when one pyrimidine ring rotates and its C4 atom forms a new bond with the C6 atom of the other ring. Both structures distort the normal structure of the DNA double helix and are highly mutagenic if left unrepaired. If present during DNA replication, UV damage leads to "UV signature" transition mutations (e.g., TT ⇨ CC) [67]. Alternatively, UV photolesions can be repaired through NER which is a multifactorial genomic stability pathway designed to identify and repair DNA damage using the undamaged sister strand as a template to ensure fidelity of process (Figure 9) [68].

Briefly, NER can begin in actively transcribed genes (TCR) when RNA polymerase stalls because of DNA damage or anywhere in the genome regardless of gene expression (GGR) through the surveillance activities of a protein complex between xeroderma pigmentosum (XP) complementation group C (XPC) and HR23B [69]. Damage recognition is followed by recruitment of the TFIIH complex which is made up of several proteins including the XPB and XPD helicases that unwind the double helix in the vicinity of the UV photolesion [70-72].

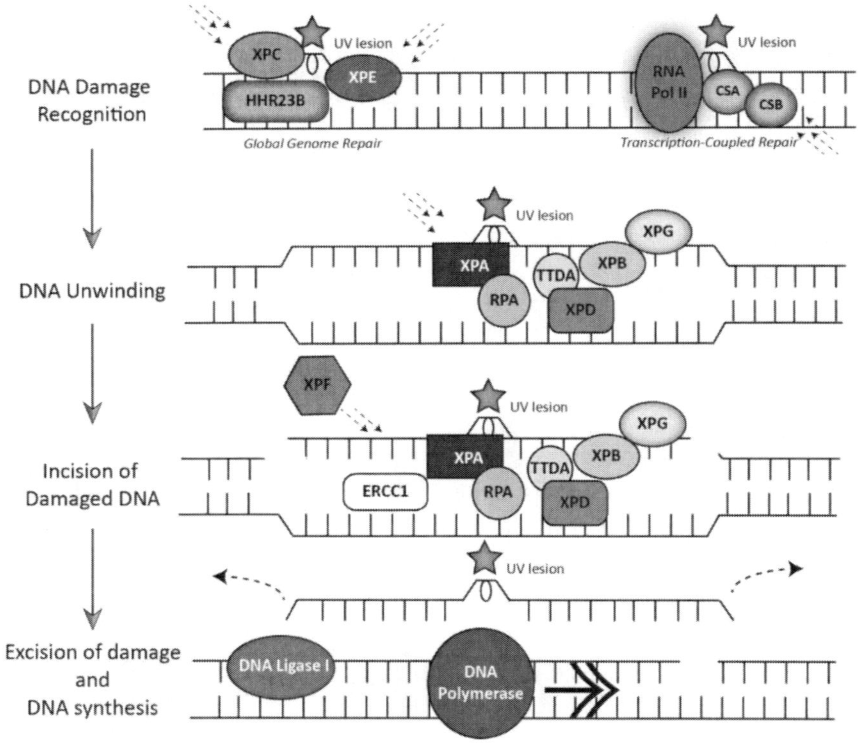

Figure 9. Nucleotide excision repair (NER). NER is a DNA repair pathway responsible for clearing helix-distorting mutagenic lesions such as UV photodimers. It is mediated by multiple proteins that work in concert to identify DNA lesions, unwind and excise a small sequence of DNA containing the damage, replace the missing region with DNA synthesis using the complementary undamaged strand for fidelity and finally to ligate newly synthesized DNA to complete repair of damage. NER can be initiated globally regardless of transcriptional activity by RNA polymerase, or in actively transcribed regions by involvement of Cockayne syndrome proteins A and B.

Once unwound, the relaxed DNA structure is stabilized by XPA and RPA, and endonucleases XPF and XPG cleave the damage strand on either side of the photolesion to remove the damaged bases and adjacent bases from the genome [73]. The resultant gap is filled in by polymerases δ and ε, using the complementary strand to direct sequence specificity. In this manner, NER is critical in reducing the frequency of UV-dependent carcinogenesis. The natural history of patients with XP, a disease caused by homozygous deficiency in any one of at least eight NER proteins is a testament to the importance of NER in UV resistance [66, 74]. Individuals affected by XP are highly sensitive to UV radiation and develop epidermal thinning, telangiectasias, and altered pigmentation early in childhood despite sun-avoidance behaviors. Furthermore, XP patients have up to a 2,000-fold increase in melanoma and other skin cancers, with malignancies diagnosed several decades earlier than sporadic cases [75].

cAMP Signaling and NER.

In whole skin or isolated melanocytes, MC1R signaling enhances the rate of clearance of UV-induced DNA photodamage by up-regulating NER. This can be measured by quantifying repair of UV photoproducts such as cyclobutane dimers (Figure 10) [33]. Using a variety of primary and transformed human melanocyte cell lines, we found a marked reduction in the time needed to repair 50% of UV damage after treating cells with the cAMP inducer forskolin (Figure 10A) [33].

Similarly, the functional importance of MC1R signaling was confirmed in HEK cells transfected with either wild type or RHC (loss-of-function) MC1R constructs. Incubation with α-MSH in these cells resulted in accelerated clearance of UV photodamage only in the presence of functional MC1R (Figure 10B) [33].

Most critically, we found that cAMP-enhanced NER reduced UV-induced mutation frequency in melanocytes, again confirming MSH effect only in the presence of functional MC1R (Figure 10C,D). Importantly, treatment of cells with forskolin could overcome MC1R loss-of-function, implying that cAMP enhancement of NER is pharmacologically rescuable (Figure 10C,D) [33].

We noted forskolin enhancement of melanocyte genomic stability in whole skin as well as in purified cell cultures [33]. Thus, using a transgenic animal model with "humanized skin", we found blunted repair of UV photoproducts when Mc1r was mutant (Figure 9E) and we noted enhancement of NER when such animals were treated with topically-applied forskolin

(Figure 9F). Therefore we concluded that manipulation of cAMP levels in the skin could impact melanocytic recovery from UV damage.

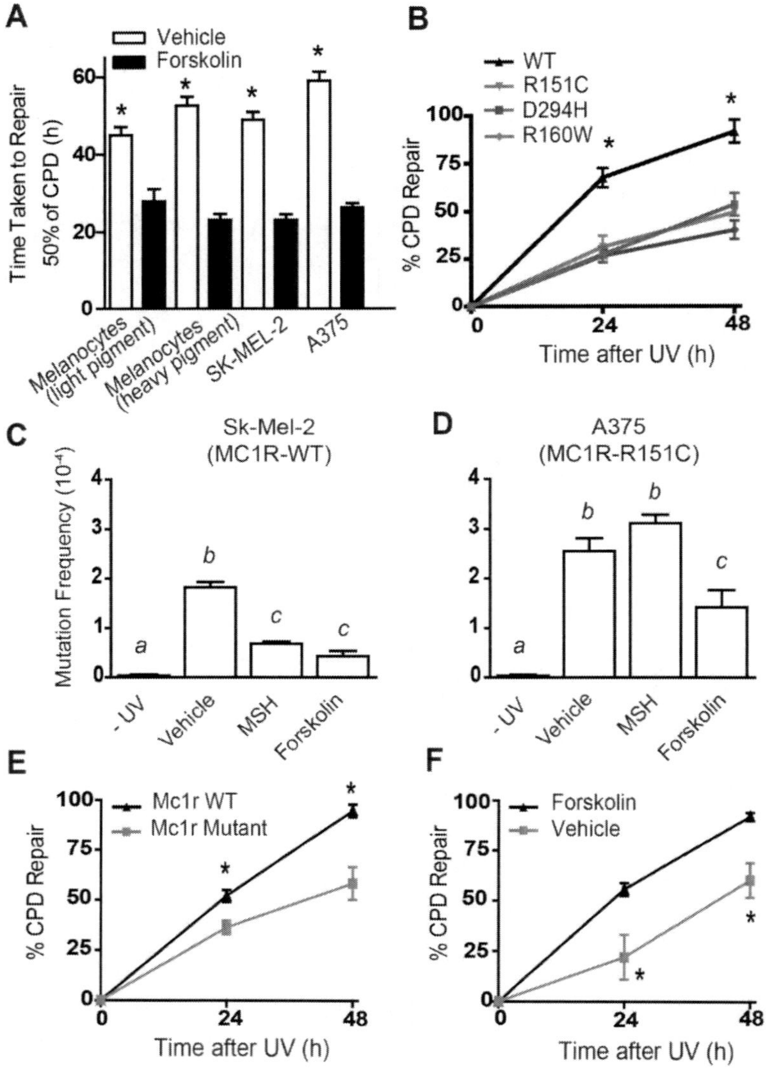

Figure 10. cAMP enhances NER and reduces mutagenesis in melanocytes. A) time needed to repair 50% of thymine dimer load in a variety of human melanocytes treated either with control or forskolin (10 uM), B) NER efficiency of HEK cells transfected with wt or RHC mutant MC1R and treated with MSH (100 nM), C,D) mutagenesis assays of MC1R wt or defective melanoma lines. Note reduced UV-induced mutation

frequency in cells after cAMP stimulation, E) NER repair efficiency in UV-exposed *K14-Scf* transgenic *Mc1r* wt or mutant (*Mc1r*$^{e/e}$) mice, F) NER enhancement by topically-applied forskolin to *K14-Scf Mc1r*$^{e/e}$ mice. All data shown with permission.

Recently, we reported the molecular mechanism by which MC1R/cAMP signaling enhances DNA repair in melanocytes. Elevating melanocytic cAMP levels, either through effective MSH-MC1R interactions or pharmacologically through forskolin-mediated adenylyl cyclase activation, causes protein kinase A (PKA) to phosphorylate the ataxia and rad3 related protein (ATR) on a specific residue (S435) which promotes its biochemical association with the NER factor XPA and directs XPA to sites of UV photodamage in nuclear DNA [33]. PKA-mediated ATR phosphorylation is essential for cAMP-enhanced NER and UV protection in melanocytes and introduces potential molecular targets (notably PKA and ATR) as relevant in melanoma prevention. Overall we conclude that MC1R signaling enhances NER and that manipulation of cAMP, for example with forskolin, promotes melanocyte genome maintenance and resistance to carcinogenesis.

Therapeutic Stimulation of Melanocyte cAMP Levels.

Various laboratories and companies are developing ways to exploit the MSH-MC1R signaling axis for clinical use. Stimulating cAMP levels in the skin is attractive for a variety of reasons:

- Increasing cAMP levels in epidermal melanocytes stimulates pigment synthesis and cutaneous deposition of melanin. To our knowledge, pharmacologic cAMP induction is not mutagenic (as opposed to UV).
- Sunless tanning would lessen the need for purposeful UV-seeking behavior among individuals desiring a darker skin complexion and would thus reduce the frequency of melanocyte mutations.
- Pharmacologically-induced melanin acts as a built-in sunblock and protects the skin against UV penetration and UV damage.
- Stimulating melanocyte cAMP levels promotes repair and clearance of UV photodamage in melanocytes. Accelerating DNA repair reduces mutation rates.
- Topical cAMP stimulation promotes epidermal thickening in mice, which itself protects the skin against UV damage.
- Increasing melanocyte cAMP levels may be a highly effective melanoma prevention strategy.

Therefore there is great interest in developing novel therapeutics to increase melanocyte cAMP levels in the skin [41]. There are three major theoretical approaches for increasing cAMP in melanocytes in the skin. The first mechanism of action is to exploit melanocortin effects on the MC1R using MSH or MSH analogues [28, 29, 76, 77]. This approach, particularly with topically-applied agents, offers the specificity of melanocyte-directed cAMP stimulation because melanocytes are thought to be the only cells in the skin that express MC1R. The limitation of MC1R-directed therapies, however, is that they would not be expected to be effective in the scenario of homozygous loss-of-function MC1R mutations. This is an important caveat because MC1R-dysfunctional individuals are at high risk for melanoma and therefore could not be helped by this approach. Thus, melanocortin-based approaches sacrifice generalizability for the sake of specificity. Other approaches rely on pharmacologic induction of adenylyl cyclase activity (e.g. by forskolin) inhibition of phosphodiesterase activity (e.g. by rolipram) to manipulate melanocyte cAMP levels irrespective of MC1R status [41-44, 78-80]. These drugs should work even in individuals with homozygous MC1R loss-of-function mutations because they pharmacologically induce cAMP in an MC1R-independent manner. In so doing, pharmacologic cAMP inducers could provide MC1R-defective individuals with UV protection and melanoma prevention. However, such agents would be expected to affect many cell types in addition to melanocytes and therefore lack the specificity of melanocortin analogues.

Before cAMP rescue can be translationally adopted, much work remains to be done to understand the usefulness and potential consequences of manipulating cAMP levels in the skin. Key hurdles to overcome are to design ways of targeting agents to melanocytes in the skin and to limit systemic exposure and unwanted off-target effects. Topical preparations offer direct application to the skin, however their efficacy may be influenced by ineffective transdermal penetration or systemic uptake of the active agent into the circulation from the skin. On the other hand, oral or injectable routing may bypass the need for a transdermal preparation however systemic effects might be greater.

CONCLUSION

Despite a clear understanding of the causative role UV exposure plays in the development of the disease and widespread public health campaigns to limit time spent in the sun or artificial tanning beds, melanoma is a growing and significant public health threat. Loss-of-function polymorphisms of MC1R signaling, which result in reduced melanocyte cAMP levels, strongly correlate with fair complexion, a tendency to burn rather than tan and an increased lifetime melanoma risk. The MC1R/cAMP signaling axis not only leads to the production of UV-protective melanin, but also enhances melanocytic ability to repair UV-damaged DNA. When applied to the skin, forskolin potently increases cutaneous cAMP levels and induces several UV-protective changes in melanocytes. By promoting melanocyte genomic stability, topical forskolin may prove to be a useful UV- and melanoma-preventive strategy.

ACKNOWLEDGMENTS

This work was supported by the following NIH grants: R01 CA131075, UL1TR000117, ES07266, T32 ES007266, and T32CA165990. We also thank the Regina Drury/Children's Miracle Network Chair in Pediatric Research Fund, the Wendy Will Case Cancer Research Fund, the Markey Cancer Foundation, the Children's Miracle Network, and the Jennifer and David Dickens Melanoma Research Foundation.

REFERENCES

[1] Elwood M, Gallagher R. Skin cancer epidemiology in 1996: the Third Symposium on the Epidemiology of Melanoma and Non-melanocytic Skin Cancer. *Melanoma Res.* 1997;7(1):74-7.

[2] Slominski A, Wortsman J. Neuroendocrinology of the skin. *Endocr Rev.* 2000;21(5):457-87.

[3] Fuchs E, Raghavan S. Getting under the skin of epidermal morphogenesis. *Nat. Rev. Genet.* 2002;3(3):199-209.

[4] Madison KC. Barrier function of the skin: "la raison d'etre" of the epidermis. *J. Invest Dermatol.* 2003;121(2):231-41.

[5] Slominski A, Fischer TW, Zmijewski MA, Wortsman J, Semak I, Zbytek B, et al. On the role of melatonin in skin physiology and pathology. *Endocrine.* 2005;27(2):137-48.

[6] Proksch E, Brandner JM, Jensen JM. The skin: an indispensable barrier. *Exp. Dermatol.* 2008;17(12):1063-72.

[7] D'Orazio J, Jarrett S, Amaro-Ortiz A, Scott T. UV Radiation and the Skin. *Int J Mol Sci.* 2013;14(6):12222-48.
[8] Slominski A, Tobin DJ, Shibahara S, Wortsman J. Melanin pigmentation in mammalian skin and its hormonal regulation. *Physiol Rev.* 2004;84(4):1155-228.
[9] Plonka PM, Passeron T, Brenner M, Tobin DJ, Shibahara S, Thomas A, et al. What are melanocytes really doing all day long...? *Exp. Dermatol.* 2009;18(9):799-819.
[10] Bristow BN, Casil J, Sorvillo F, Basurto-Davila R, Kuo T. Melanoma-related mortality and productivity losses in the USA, 1990-2008. *Melanoma Res.* 2013;23(4):331-5.
[11] Marks R. Epidemiology of melanoma. *Clin. Exp. Dermatol.* 2000;25(6):459-63.
[12] Schulman JM, Fisher DE. Indoor ultraviolet tanning and skin cancer: health risks and opportunities. *Curr. Opin. Oncol.* 2009;21(2):144-9.
[13] Boniol M, Autier P, Boyle P, Gandini S. Cutaneous melanoma attributable to sunbed use: systematic review and meta-analysis. *BMJ.* 2012;345:e4757.
[14] Kubica AW, Brewer JD. Melanoma in immunosuppressed patients. Mayo Clin Proc. 2012;87(10):991-1003.
[15] Goldstein AM, Tucker MA. Dysplastic nevi and melanoma. *Cancer Epidemiol Biomarkers Prev.* 2013;22(4):528-32.
[16] Usher-Smith JA, Emery J, Kassianos AP, Walter FM. Risk prediction models for melanoma: a systematic review. *Cancer Epidemiol Biomarkers Prev.* 2014;23(8):1450-63.
[17] Vuong K, McGeechan K, Armstrong BK, Cust AE. Risk prediction models for incident primary cutaneous melanoma: a systematic review. *JAMA Dermatol.* 2014;150(4):434-44.
[18] Prota G. Melanins, melanogenesis and melanocytes: looking at their functional significance from the chemist's viewpoint. *Pigment Cell Res.* 2000;13(4):283-93.
[19] Scherer D, Kumar R. Genetics of pigmentation in skin cancer--a review. *Mutat Res.* 2010;705(2):141-53.
[20] Wood JM, Gibbons NC, Schallreuter KU. Melanocortins in human melanocytes. *Cell Mol Biol* (Noisy-le-grand). 2006;52(2):75-8.
[21] Garcia-Borron JC, Abdel-Malek Z, Jimenez-Cervantes C. MC1R, the cAMP pathway, and the response to solar UV: extending the horizon beyond pigmentation. *Pigment cell & melanoma research.* 2014;27(5):699-720.

[22] Nasti TH, Timares L. MC1R, Eumelanin and Pheomelanin: their role in determining the susceptibility to skin cancer. *Photochem Photobiol.* 2014.

[23] Yamaguchi Y, Brenner M, Hearing VJ. The regulation of skin pigmentation. *J. Biol Chem.* 2007;282(38):27557-61.

[24] Lin JY, Fisher DE. Melanocyte biology and skin pigmentation. *Nature.* 2007;445(7130):843-50.

[25] Lamason RL, Mohideen MA, Mest JR, Wong AC, Norton HL, Aros MC, et al. SLC24A5, a putative cation exchanger, affects pigmentation in zebrafish and humans. *Science.* 2005;310(5755):1782-6.

[26] Abdel-Malek Z, Suzuki I, Tada A, Im S, Akcali C. The melanocortin-1 receptor and human pigmentation. *Ann N Y Acad Sci.* 1999;885:117-33.

[27] Rouzaud F, Hearing VJ. Regulatory elements of the melanocortin 1 receptor. *Peptides.* 2005;26(10):1858-70.

[28] Abdel-Malek ZA, Swope VB, Starner RJ, Koikov L, Cassidy P, Leachman S. Melanocortins and the melanocortin 1 receptor, moving translationally towards melanoma prevention. *Arch. Biochem. Biophys.* 2014.

[29] Abdel-Malek ZA, Ruwe A, Kavanagh-Starner R, Kadekaro AL, Swope V, Haskell-Luevano C, et al. alpha-MSH tripeptide analogs activate the melanocortin 1 receptor and reduce UV-induced DNA damage in human melanocytes. *Pigment cell & melanoma research.* 2009;22(5):635-44.

[30] Kadekaro AL, Chen J, Yang J, Chen S, Jameson J, Swope VB, et al. Alpha-melanocyte-stimulating hormone suppresses oxidative stress through a p53-mediated signaling pathway in human melanocytes. *Mol. Cancer Res.* 2012;10(6):778-86.

[31] Wong SS, Ainger SA, Leonard JH, Sturm RA. MC1R variant allele effects on UVR-induced phosphorylation of p38, p53, and DDB2 repair protein responses in melanocytic cells in culture. *J. Invest Dermatol.* 2012;132(5):1452-61.

[32] Swope V, Alexander C, Starner R, Schwemberger S, Babcock G, Abdel-Malek ZA. Significance of the melanocortin 1 receptor in the DNA damage response of human melanocytes to ultraviolet radiation. *Pigment cell & melanoma research.* 2014;27(4):601-10.

[33] Jarrett SG, Horrell EM, Christian PA, Vanover JC, Boulanger MC, Zou Y, et al. PKA-mediated phosphorylation of ATR promotes recruitment of XPA to UV-induced DNA damage. *Mol Cell.* 2014;54(6):999-1011.

[34] April CS, Barsh GS. Distinct pigmentary and melanocortin 1 receptor-dependent components of cutaneous defense against ultraviolet radiation. *PLoS Genet.* 2007;3(1):e9.
[35] Song X, Mosby N, Yang J, Xu A, Abdel-Malek Z, Kadekaro AL. alpha-MSH activates immediate defense responses to UV-induced oxidative stress in human melanocytes. *Pigment cell & melanoma research.* 2009;22(6):809-18.
[36] Henri P, Beaumel S, Guezennec A, Poumes C, Stoebner PE, Stasia MJ, et al. MC1R expression in HaCaT keratinocytes inhibits UVA-induced ROS production via NADPH oxidase- and cAMP-dependent mechanisms. *J. Cell Physiol.* 2012;227(6):2578-85.
[37] Mitra D, Luo X, Morgan A, Wang J, Hoang MP, Lo J, et al. An ultraviolet-radiation-independent pathway to melanoma carcinogenesis in the red hair/fair skin background. *Nature.* 2012;491(7424):449-53.
[38] Suzuki I, Cone RD, Im S, Nordlund J, Abdel-Malek ZA. Binding of melanotropic hormones to the melanocortin receptor MC1R on human melanocytes stimulates proliferation and melanogenesis. *Endocrinology.* 1996;137(5):1627-33.
[39] Suzuki I, Tada A, Ollmann MM, Barsh GS, Im S, Lamoreux ML, et al. Agouti signaling protein inhibits melanogenesis and the response of human melanocytes to alpha-melanotropin. *J. Invest Dermatol.* 1997;108(6):838-42.
[40] Suzuki I, Im S, Tada A, Scott C, Akcali C, Davis MB, et al. Participation of the melanocortin-1 receptor in the UV control of pigmentation. *J. Investig Dermatol Symp Proc.* 1999;4(1):29-34.
[41] D'Orazio JA, Nobuhisa T, Cui R, Arya M, Spry M, Wakamatsu K, et al. Topical drug rescue strategy and skin protection based on the role of Mc1r in UV-induced tanning. *Nature.* 2006;443(7109):340-4.
[42] Spry ML, Vanover JC, Scott T, Abona-Ama O, Wakamatsu K, Ito S, et al. Prolonged treatment of fair-skinned mice with topical forskolin causes persistent tanning and UV protection. *Pigment cell & melanoma research.* 2009;22(2):219-29.
[43] Khaled M, Levy C, Fisher DE. Control of melanocyte differentiation by a MITF-PDE4D3 homeostatic circuit. *Genes Dev.* 2010;24(20):2276-81.
[44] Amaro-Ortiz A, Vanover JC, Scott TL, D'Orazio JA. Pharmacologic induction of epidermal melanin and protection against sunburn in a humanized mouse model. *J. Vis. Exp.* 2013(79).
[45] Hadley ME, Haskell-Luevano C. The proopiomelanocortin system. *Ann. N Y Acad Sci.* 1999;885:1-21.

[46] Cui R, Widlund HR, Feige E, Lin JY, Wilensky DL, Igras VE, et al. Central role of p53 in the suntan response and pathologic hyperpigmentation. *Cell.* 2007;128(5):853-64.

[47] Kadekaro AL, Kanto H, Kavanagh R, Abdel-Malek Z. Significance of the melanocortin 1 receptor in regulating human melanocyte pigmentation, proliferation, and survival. *Ann. N Y Acad Sci.* 2003;994:359-65.

[48] Hida T, Wakamatsu K, Sviderskaya EV, Donkin AJ, Montoliu L, Lynn Lamoreux M, et al. Agouti protein, mahogunin, and attractin in pheomelanogenesis and melanoblast-like alteration of melanocytes: a cAMP-independent pathway. *Pigment cell & melanoma research.* 2009;22(5):623-34.

[49] Candille SI, Kaelin CB, Cattanach BM, Yu B, Thompson DA, Nix MA, et al. A -defensin mutation causes black coat color in domestic dogs. *Science.* 2007;318(5855):1418-23.

[50] Swope VB, Jameson JA, McFarland KL, Supp DM, Miller WE, McGraw DW, et al. Defining MC1R regulation in human melanocytes by its agonist alpha-melanocortin and antagonists agouti signaling protein and beta-defensin 3. *J. Invest Dermatol.* 2012;132(9):2255-62.

[51] Kunisada T, Lu SZ, Yoshida H, Nishikawa S, Nishikawa S, Mizoguchi M, et al. Murine cutaneous mastocytosis and epidermal melanocytosis induced by keratinocyte expression of transgenic stem cell factor. *J. Exp. Med.* 1998;187(10):1565-73.

[52] Phung B, Sun J, Schepsky A, Steingrimsson E, Ronnstrand L. C-KIT signaling depends on microphthalmia-associated transcription factor for effects on cell proliferation. *PLoS One*. 2011;6(8):e24064.

[53] Wu M, Hemesath TJ, Takemoto CM, Horstmann MA, Wells AG, Price ER, et al. c-Kit triggers dual phosphorylations, which couple activation and degradation of the essential melanocyte factor Mi. *Genes Dev.* 2000;14(3):301-12.

[54] Patel MB. Forskolin: a successful therapeutic phytomolecule. *East and Central African Journal of Pharmaceutical Sciences*. 2010;13:25-32.

[55] Geller AI, During MJ, Haycock JW, Freese A, Neve R. Long-term increases in neurotransmitter release from neuronal cells expressing a constitutively active adenylate cyclase from a herpes simplex virus type 1 vector. *Proc. Natl. Acad. Sci. USA*. 1993;90(16):7603-7.

[56] da Conceicao AO, de Oliveira FF, de Oliveira RA, de JdSJA, Takser L, Reyes-Moreno C, et al. Lantana macrophylla Schauer (Verbenaceae) ethanolic extract induces activation of ERK1/2 and p38 MAPKs

pathway and Ca2+ imbalance in human trophoblasts derived cell lines. *Food Chem Toxicol.* 2012;50(3-4):1001-12.

[57] Doseyici S, Mehmetoglu I, Toker A, Yerlikaya FH, Erbay E. The effects of forskolin and rolipram on cAMP, cGMP and free fatty acid levels in diet induced obesity. *Biotech Histochem.* 2014;89(5):388-92.

[58] Enomoto M, Jain A, Pan J, Shifrin Y, Van Vliet T, McNamara PJ, et al. Newborn rat response to single vs. combined cGMP-dependent pulmonary vasodilators. *Am. J. Physiol. Lung Cell Mol. Physiol.* 2014;306(2):L207-15.

[59] Galeotti N, Ghelardini C, Zoppi M, Del Bene E, Raimondi L, Beneforti E, et al. Hypofunctionality of Gi proteins as aetiopathogenic mechanism for migraine and cluster headache. *Cephalalgia.* 2001;21(1):38-45.

[60] Onoue H, Katusic ZS. The effect of subarachnoid hemorrhage on mechanisms of vasodilation mediated by cyclic adenosine monophosphate. *J. Neurosurg.* 1998;89(1):111-7.

[61] Cumbay MG, Watts VJ. Novel regulatory properties of human type 9 adenylate cyclase. *J. Pharmacol. Exp Ther.* 2004;310(1):108-15.

[62] Chen J, Hammell DC, Spry M, D'Orazio JA, Stinchcomb AL. In vitro skin diffusion study of pure forskolin versus a forskolin-containing Plectranthus barbatus root extract. *J. Nat. Prod.* 2009;72(4):769-71.

[63] Vanover JC, Spry ML, Hamilton L, Wakamatsu K, Ito S, D'Orazio JA. Stem cell factor rescues tyrosinase expression and pigmentation in discreet anatomic locations in albino mice. *Pigment cell & melanoma research.* 2009;22(6):827-38.

[64] Ura K, Hayes JJ. Nucleotide excision repair and chromatin remodeling. *Eur. J. Biochem.* 2002;269(9):2288-93.

[65] Ichihashi M, Ueda M, Budiyanto A, Bito T, Oka M, Fukunaga M, et al. UV-induced skin damage. *Toxicology.* 2003;189(1-2):21-39.

[66] Bergoglio V, Magnaldo T. Nucleotide excision repair and related human diseases. *Genome Dyn.* 2006;1:35-52.

[67] Wallin H. A molecular pathway for UV-induced CC to TT mutations. *Mutat Res.* 2000;447(2):317-8.

[68] Eller MS, Ostrom K, Gilchrest BA. DNA damage enhances melanogenesis. *Proc. Natl. Acad. Sci. USA.* 1996;93(3):1087-92.

[69] Tremblay M, Toussaint M, D'Amours A, Conconi A. Nucleotide excision repair and photolyase repair of UV photoproducts in nucleosomes: assessing the existence of nucleosome and non-nucleosome rDNA chromatin in vivo. *Biochem Cell Biol.* 2009;87(1):337-46.

[70] Novarina D, Amara F, Lazzaro F, Plevani P, Muzi-Falconi M. Mind the gap: keeping UV lesions in check. *DNA Repair* (Amst). 2011;10(7): 751-9.

[71] Palomera-Sanchez Z, Zurita M. Open, repair and close again: chromatin dynamics and the response to UV-induced DNA damage. *DNA Repair* (Amst). 2011;10(2):119-25.

[72] Reed SH. Nucleotide excision repair in chromatin: damage removal at the drop of a HAT. *DNA Repair* (Amst). 2011;10(7):734-42.

[73] Rastogi RP, Richa, Kumar A, Tyagi MB, Sinha RP. Molecular mechanisms of ultraviolet radiation-induced DNA damage and repair. *J. Nucleic Acids.* 2010;2010:592980.

[74] Kraemer KH, DiGiovanna JJ. Xeroderma Pigmentosum. In: Pagon RA, Adam MP, Ardinger HH, Bird TD, Dolan CR, Fong CT, et al., editors. *Gene Reviews*(R). Seattle (WA)1993.

[75] DiGiovanna JJ, Kraemer KH. Shining a light on xeroderma pigmentosum. *J. Invest Dermatol.* 2012;132(3 Pt 2):785-96.

[76] Haskell-Luevano C, Shenderovich MD, Sharma SD, Nikiforovich GV, Hadley ME, Hruby VJ. Design, synthesis, biology, and conformations of bicyclic alpha-melanotropin analogues. *J. Med. Chem.* 1995;38(10):1736-50.

[77] Abdel-Malek ZA. Development of alpha-melanocortin analogs for melanoma prevention and targeting. *Adv. Exp. Med. Biol.* 2010;681:126-32.

[78] Passeron T, Namiki T, Passeron HJ, Le Pape E, Hearing VJ. Forskolin protects keratinocytes from UVB-induced apoptosis and increases DNA repair independent of its effects on melanogenesis. *J. Invest Dermatol.* 2009;129(1):162-6.

[79] Scott TL, Christian PA, Kesler MV, Donohue KM, Shelton B, Wakamatsu K, et al. Pigment-independent cAMP-mediated epidermal thickening protects against cutaneous UV injury by keratinocyte proliferation. *Exp. Dermatol.* 2012;21(10):771-7.

[80] Amaro-Ortiz A, Yan B, D'Orazio JA. Ultraviolet radiation, aging and the skin: prevention of damage by topical cAMP manipulation. *Molecules.* 2014;19(5):6202-19.

In: Forskolin
Editor: Marty H. Walker

ISBN: 978-1-63463-918-7

Chapter 2

Oral Administration of Forskolin Decreases Retinal Damage after Experimental Induction of Ocular Hypertension in the Rat

Nicola Pescosolido[1], Gianfranco Scarsella[2] and Dario Rusciano[3,*,#]
[1]Dipartimento di Scienze Cardiovascolari, Respiratorie, Nefrologiche, Anestesiologiche e Geriatriche, Sapienza - Università di Roma, Roma, Italy
[2]Dipartimento di Biologia e Biotecnologie "Charles Darwin", Sapienza - Università di Roma, Roma, Italy
[3]Sooft italia SpA, Roma, Italy

Abstract

Purpose: The aim of the present work was to show the potential neuroprotective activity of forskolin, a receptor-independent activator of

---

* Corresponding author: Dario Rusciano, Sooft italia SpA, Via Salvatore Quasimodo 136, 00144 Roma, Italy. Email: dario.rusciano@sooft.it phone +3906 83766253; fax +3906 83766793.

Proprietary interests: G. Scarsella (none); N. Pescosolido (none); D. Rusciano (is a full time employee of Sooft Italia, an Italian pharmaceutical company that produces a food supplement containing forskolin).

adenylate-cyclase, in an experimental model of ocular hypertension in the rat.

Methods: Methylcellulose at 2% was injected into the anterior chamber of rat eyes to induce IOP elevation. Animals were either treated or not with forskolin (1 mg/Kg) in their diet.

Results: Seven days after IOP elevation, rat retinas were evaluated for apoptosis (TUNEL and caspase 3) and iNOS. Forskolin treatment resulted in a reduced increase of IOP after methylcellulose injection, and a decreased production of iNOS, that resulted in a reduced expression of caspase 3 and TUNEL positive cells.

Conclusion: The combined action on IOP and neuron survival suggests a neuroprotective activity of forskolin in glaucomatous neurodegenerative disease, in which elevated IOP is the main risk factor, but not the only determinant of the progressive death of retinal ganglion cells.

Keywords: Glaucoma, IOP, forskolin, neuroprotection, neurotrophins

INTRODUCTION

Primary open angle glaucoma (POAG) is a progressive degenerative disease of the optic nerve [1] and the second leading cause of blindness in the world, affecting roughly 67 million people globally [2]. One of the main risk factors for glaucoma is high intraocular pressure (IOP), which may rise above statistically normal values. This increase can be ascribed, from a strictly physical point of view, to a defective efflux of the aqueous humor from the anterior chamber of the eye [3]. A common feature of POAG involves an excavation of the optic disk, which is extended to its margins, thus increasing the cup-to-disk ratio. Several studies indicate that early lesions occur in the optic nerve at the level of the lamina cribrosa [4]. Intraocular hypertension may cause significant overexpression of caspase 3 in retinal ganglion cells (RGCs), which is a commonly accepted marker of programmed cell death [5-6], further supporting the neurodegenerative nature of POAG. In fact, decreasing IOP appears to be a necessary, although not sufficient, strategy to prevent glaucoma progression, which is due to the continuous deterioration of RGCs that evidently can occur and continue also in the presence of a normal or normalized IOP [7-8]. Therefore, nowadays glaucoma is considered to be a neurological disease, an optic neuropathy for which ocular hypertension is the main risk factor, but not necessarily the primary causative agent [9].

This concept is further corroborated by the recent finding reported by Grieshaber and Flammer [10]: comparison by metanalysis of the effects of two beta-blockers shows that 'despite a similar IOP reduction, patients treated with betaxolol had a smaller rate of visual field deterioration than patients treated with timolol'. The Authors conclude against the dogma stating that "the greater the IOP reduction the better the visual field prognosis", suggesting that also the nature of the drug by which IOP reduction is achieved is important. In fact, betaxolol has also been shown to have neuroprotective activities, improving ocular blood flow [11], and protecting RGCs from apoptosis [12-13]. Moreover, a very recent paper published by Krupin and colleagues [14] shows that in a group of patients with low tension POAG treated with either timolol or brimonidine, despite a similar response to the hypotensive activity of each drug, the patients treated with brimonidine (a supposed neuroprotective agent) progressed (by visual field analysis) at a much slower rate during 30 months of observation than those treated with timolol. These data confirm that IOP decrease and neuroprotection can be two different, albeit concurrent, events.

Forskolin (7beta-acetoxy-8, 13-epoxy-1a, 6β, 9a-trihydroxy-labd-14-en-11-one) is a diterpenoid isolated from the plant *Coleus forskohlii* (Lamiaceae). In India, since ancient times, *Coleus forskohlii* has been used in traditional Hindu and Ayurvedic medicine [15]. It was recorded in the ancient Sanskrit texts that *Coleus forskohlii* was used as a medicinal herb to treat hypertension, congestive heart failure, eczema, colic, respiratory disorders, painful urination, insomnia, convulsions, asthma, angina, psoriasis and for prevention of cancer metastases [16-18]. Forskolin is a receptor-independent adenylate-cyclase activator, so that the concentration of the second-messenger cAMP rapidly increases in forskolin-stimulated cells [19-20]. Of the 9 types of adenylate-cyclase in humans, forskolin can activate all but type IX, which is found in spermatozoa [21]. Human non pigmented ciliary epithelial cells have been shown to contain adenylate-cyclase (subtypes II, IV), and bovine trabecular meshwork cells contain subtype VII, the activity of which contributes to the regulation of aqueous humour dynamics [22-23]. Elevation of cAMP after forskolin treatment apparently activates a reverse flow of secretion in the ciliary body, from the posterior chamber into the stroma, which counteracts the normal flow of secretion, proceeding from the stroma into the posterior chamber. This results in a decreased net inflow of aqueous humour into the eye chambers [24-25]. Moreover, it has been described that elevation of cAMP inhibits the activation of the Rho protein, thus causing a disorganization of the actin cytoskeleton, which in the trabecular meshwork has been shown to result in tissue relaxation, and an increase of AH outflow [26-27]. The combination of these two events may explain the hypotensive effect of topical administration of forskolin, as shown in experimental animals and humans [28-29]. Moreover, forskolin-mediated activation of cAMP contributes to neuronal cell survival and growth [30].

Therefore, we set out to establish a proof of concept on the neuroprotective ability of forskolin in an experimental rat model system of retinal ischemia, simulating the high IOP damage that may occur in hypertensive glaucoma.

Materials and Methods

Animals, Treatments, and Experimental Procedures

All experimental procedures were in accordance with the ARVO Statement for the Use of Animals in Ophthalmic and Vision Research, the guidelines of the European Communities Council Directive of 24 November 1986 (86/609/EEC), Italian Health Ministry guidelines, and EU Directive 2010/63/EU for animal experiments, and were approved by the Institutional Review Board. The experimental model of ocular hypertension used in this study has been described by Zhu & Cai [31]. This model is based on inoculation with methylcellulose 2% (MTC) in the anterior chamber of a rabbit eye. MTC is a molecule capable of mechanically blocking the outflow of aqueous humour, thus leading to ocular hypertension.

Starting 7 days before IOP elevation, a group of 24 young adult rats (2-6 months old) was fed with a diet which was the same each day, either supplemented with forskolin (10 mg/Kg of an extract titrated at 10% in forskolin) or not. The treatment dose was arbitrarily chosen to be 5 times higher than the oral dose given to humans (0.2 mg/Kg) by means of a food supplement commercially available in Italy (Kronek®, Sooft italia SpA). Rats were hosted one per cage in order to control each day that they had taken the whole daily amount of food and forskolin supplement. After local anaesthesia by administration of eye drops with 0.4% oxybuprocaine (Novesine, Novartis, Basel, Switzerland), animals were slowly injected in the anterior chamber of the right eye with 15 μl of MTC 2% (SIGMA-Aldrich, St. Louis, MO, USA) in physiological solution. The IOP was monitored by a tonometer (Tonopen XL, Automated Ophthalmics, Ellicott City, MD, USA) with a measurement range between 5 and 80 mmHg. The degree of animal suffering was evaluated by the behavioural Irwin test and by the recovery of body weight [32]. Ocular inflammation was assessed by the Draize test adapted to the rat [33]. Ocular hypertension reached a maximum of 55-60 mmHg within 3-6 h after injection, and then stabilized within 24h at intermediate values around 25-30 mmHg. This method closely recalls clinical and histopathological events occurring in human glaucoma [33-35]. Seven days after the intraocular injection, animals were given general anaesthesia by intra-peritoneal injection of 500 μl sodium-thiopental solution (Farmotal, Pharmacia & Upjohn, USA) in phosphate buffered saline (PBS). They were then killed by carotid bleeding, after which the eyeballs were removed.

Histo-Morphological and Molecular Analysis

After eye enucleation, corneas were rapidly cut vertically, and the crystalline lens and vitreous humour removed. The following procedures on the residual tissues were then carried out:

- fixation in paraformaldehyde 4% for 6 h at 4°C;
- rapid wash with PBS;
- immersion in a 30% sucrose solution in PBS at 4°C overnight;
- inclusion in Killik embedding medium (Bio-Optica, Milan, Italy) then cryostat cut into 10 μm sections, horizontally, to allow longitudinal observation of the optic nerve. The sections were placed on microscope slides and stored at -20°C.

Fluorescence Immunolocalization

This method was used to localize the inducible form of the enzyme that synthesizes nitric oxide (iNOS). To detect its expression, a rabbit primary polyclonal anti-iNOS antibody (Santa Cruz) was diluted to 1:50, while the secondary antibody used was a goat anti-rabbit IgG Alexa Fluor (Molecular Probes) that is green-fluorescing. The sections, left to dry at room temperature for 30 min, were subjected to various treatments:

- washed in PBS for 5 min;
- post-fixation with alcohol at increasing volumes (70°, 95°, 100°) for 2 min;
- washed in PBS for 5 min; blocked with serum (Normal Rabbit or Goat Serum: NRS, NGS), 10% in PBS, 1 h in a moist chamber; incubation with the primary antibody diluted in PBS + BSA 1% for 1h;
- fast washed in PBS;
- incubation with the secondary antibody diluted 1:200 in PBS + 1% NGS, for 30 min at room temperature;
- washed in PBS for 5 min;
- mounting of the slides with Eukitt.

The observations were made under a fluorescence microscope and pictures taken by computerized image acquisition.

Western Blotting and Immunodetection

Western blotting was used to evaluate the expression of caspase-3, and the results normalized towards actin. The Bradford assay was used to estimate the concentration of proteins.

Preparation of protein extracts: After weighing rat retinas, they were immersed in lysis buffer (5 M urea, 2 M thiourea, 2% (w/v) CHAPS, 2% (w/v) SB 3-10, 40 mM Tris, 0.2% (w/v) Bio-Lyte 3/10, 2 mM TBP, 1 mM PMSF, and 200 μg/ml DNase I) to extract the proteins. The test-tubes were kept for 10 min. on ice, then centrifuged at 13000 rpm for 5 sec. and transferred back to ice for another 10 min. Finally, they were centrifuged for 10 min. at 13000 rpm. This procedure removed nucleic acids and debris. This last supernatant was finally collected and proteins resolved by SDS-PAGE according to Laemmli [36].

Transfer of proteins to nitrocellulose: The transfer took place by pressing the gel against a nitrocellulose filter and subjecting it to a constant electric field of 300 mA in a specifically designed chamber (BioRad). The filter was then washed with Tris-buffered saline/0.1% Tween (TBS-T) and after saturation of nonspecific bonds (TBS-T + 5% milk), the proteins were probed with the primary antibody capable of specifically detecting those of interest. During incubation, each antibody was added to a solution of TBS-T and 5%

dry milk for 1 h. After several washes with TBS-T, carried out following the absorption of the primary antibody, incubation with the secondary antibody was performed. The secondary antibodies used for caspase-3 (anti-rabbit IgG, Jackson) and actin (anti-goat IgG, Jackson) were used at a dilution of 1:5000. Finally, detection by chemiluminescence (ECL) was performed.

TUNEL Assay

At an advanced stage of the apoptosis cascade, the cell presents extensive DNA degradation which leads to the production of fragments 180-200 bp, and their multiples, in length. The *in situ* DNA fragments are highlighted by fluorescent nucleotide conjugation using the TUNEL (Terminal deoxynucleotidyl transferase mediated dUTP Nick End Labelling) technique, which consists of *in situ* labelling of DNA fragments by fluoresceinated nucleotide conjugation using terminal deoxynucleotidyl transferase.

Tissue sections with a thickness of 10 μm were subjected to DNA terminal staining using nucleotides linked to the fluorescent chromophore fluorescein. Nuclei with degraded DNA showed greater fluorescence than nuclei in which the degenerative process was absent, because the terminal transferase specifically incorporates fluorescent nucleotides onto the free 3'OH ends of fragmented DNA. The sections, left to dry at room temperature for 30 min, were subjected to the following treatments:

- rehydration through a descending alcohol series (100°, 95°, 75°; 2 min each);
- incubation with 20 μg/mL protease in 0.1% Triton X-100 at 37°C for 30 min;
- washed with PBS for 2 min;
- incubation with the TUNEL reagent (In Situ Cell Death Detection Kit, AP/ROCHE), containing 1/10 volume of terminal deoxynucleotidyl transferase and the remaining fraction of nucleotides labelled with a fluorescent chromophore, 10 μl per section at 37°C for 1 h.

On each slide, one of the sections was always used as the negative control, i.e. incubated without terminal transferase in the presence of nucleotides in order to detect any non-specific staining of the sections;

- wash with PBS for 5 min;
- slide mounting with Eukitt.

The observations were made under a fluorescence microscope and pictures taken by computerized image acquisition.

Statistical Analysis

All determinations were repeated at least four times. ANOVA test was used to compare data at different times within the same group, while Student's t-test was employed to compare data at the same time point between two different groups. P-values <0.05 were considered significant.

RESULTS

Forskolin Attenuates MTC Effects on IOP

Twenty-four young adult rats were divided into three groups: 4 animals served as normal controls; the other 20 were scheduled to receive MTC injections in the anterior ocular chamber. Of these, 10 received oral forskolin treatment (1 mg/Kg of forskolin) starting 7 days before MTC inoculation, and 10 served as forskolin-untreated controls. IOP in all groups was measured daily (always in the morning at 9:00 a.m.) for 7 days. Results shown in Figure 1 indicate that in forskolin-treated animals there is a progressive IOP decrease during the first 48 h, and a further stabilization at values around 30% below the normal in the next days, thus confirming the IOP lowering effect of orally given forskolin.

These animals were then subjected to MTC injection in the anterior chamber, and their IOP was monitored for another week. Figure 2A shows the effects of MTC injection during the first 24 h: in the first 5 min (as a consequence of the AH volume increase after the injection) there was a sudden transient elevation of IOP, reaching values of 60 mm Hg, then decreasing to normal within 1 h (Figure 2A, inset). A second peak at 55 mm Hg was reached between 1 and 3 h (the consequence of trabecular tissue clogging by MTC), lasting until 6 h, after which a steady IOP was maintained until 24 h and for the next 5 days (Figure 2B). Figure 2B also shows the different behavior of forskolin treated vs. untreated animals.

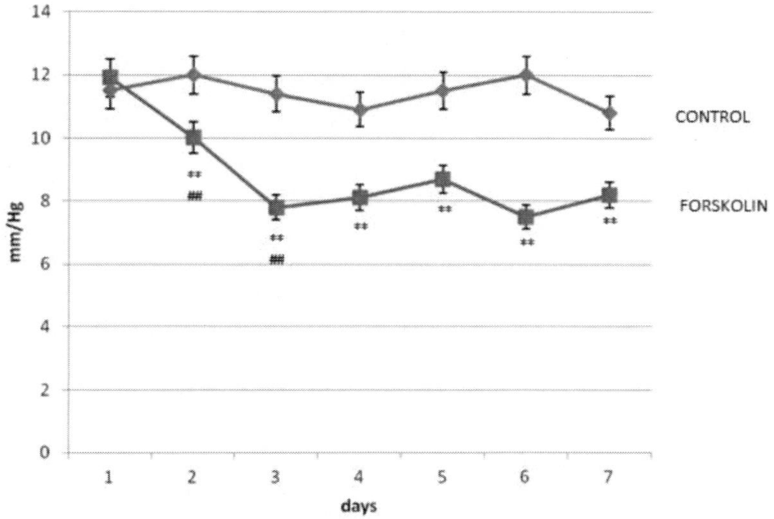

Figure 1. Oral forskolin effects on the IOP of young adult rats. A group of 24 young rats (2-6 months old) was fed with a diet which was the same each day, either supplemented with forskolin (10 mg/Kg of an extract titrated at 10% in forskolin) or not. IOP was measured each morning by a Tonopen. Average values of ten measurements ± standard error are reported. ** = p < 0.01 vs. control. ## = p < 0.01 vs. time 0.

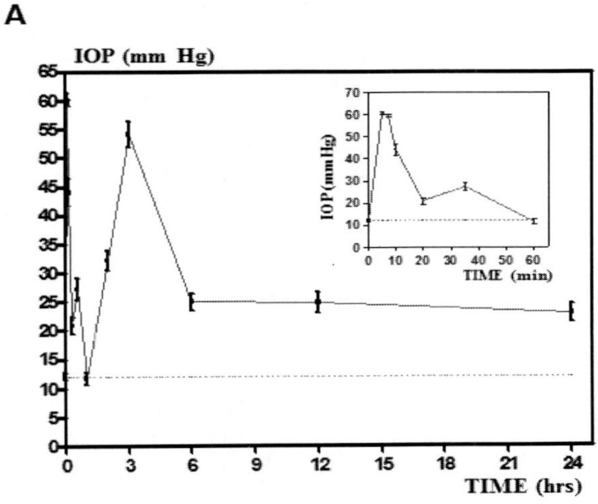

Figure 2. (Continued).

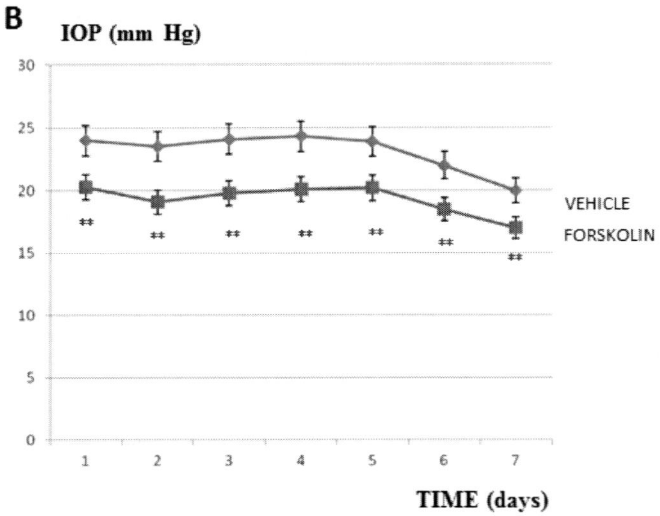

Figure 2. IOP evaluation during the first 24 hours after injection of 15 µl of MTC in the anterior chamber (continuous line). A. Baseline IOP (dotted line). Inset: Close up on the IOP variations during the first hour after MTC injection. B. Weekly trend of IOP in animals injected with MTC and treated (squares) or not (circles) with oral forskolin. Standard error bars are indicated per each point (10 determinations per point). ** = $p < 0.01$ vs. vehicle.

In fact, the steady state of IOP was reached at around 24 mm Hg for the untreated animals, whereas it was at around 20 mm Hg for forskolin fed animals. After the 5th day, a further decrease of IOP was observed in both groups of animals, however, still conserving the difference between treated and untreated.

After 7 days from the injection, the twenty retinas of each group of 10 animals (plus or minus forskolin treatment) were then analyzed (4 replicates per each analysis) for biochemical and histological markers.

Forskolin Blunts Apoptosis

Apoptotic DNA degradation in the retina can be studied using the TUNEL assay. This technique labels the nuclei of apoptotic cells in an advanced stage of death, when endonucleases have cut their DNA into defined fragments.

Figure 3 shows that 7 days after MTC injection, in forskolin-untreated animals (B) there is an intense fluorescence in the ganglion cell layer (GCL), indicating massive cell death. However, if animals were fed a forskolin diet, the fluorescence in this layer was definitely less intense, indicating a lower amount of dying cells, and a protective activity of forskolin treatment (C). Normal control retinas (A) showed no staining at all.

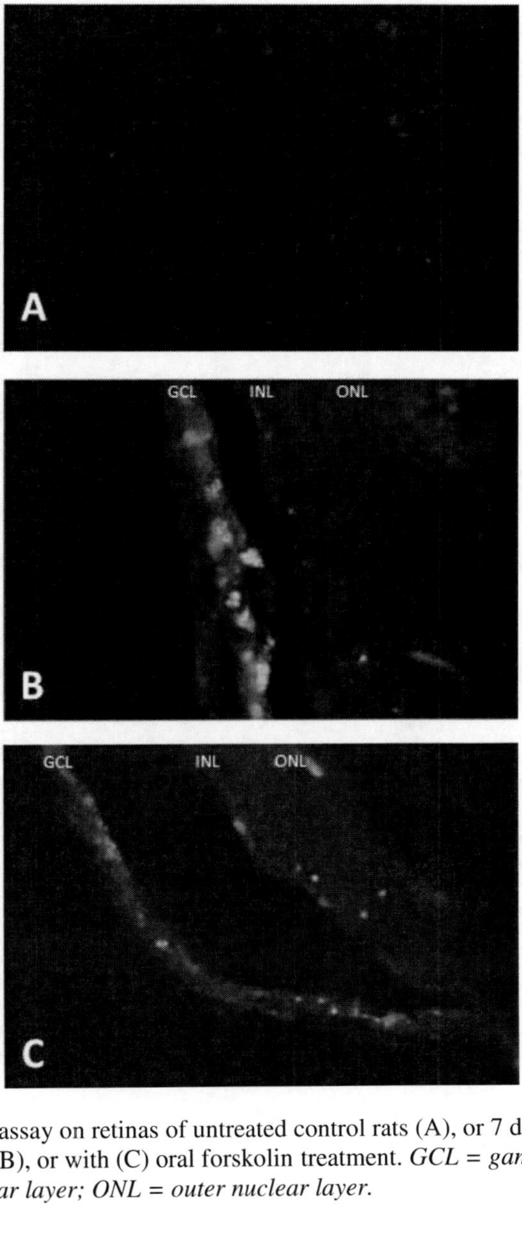

Figure 3. TUNEL assay on retinas of untreated control rats (A), or 7 days after MTC injection without (B), or with (C) oral forskolin treatment. *GCL = ganglion cell layer; INL = inner nuclear layer; ONL = outer nuclear layer.*

Forskolin Decreases iNOS Expression

iNOS is one of the main enzymes that is induced in cases of ischemic damage [37]. Similarly to what was observed with the TUNEL assay, animals treated with MTC alone showed high iNOS expression in the GCL (Figure 4A). Treatment with oral forskolin decreased iNOS expression in such layer, suggesting protection from the ischemic damage (Figure 4B).

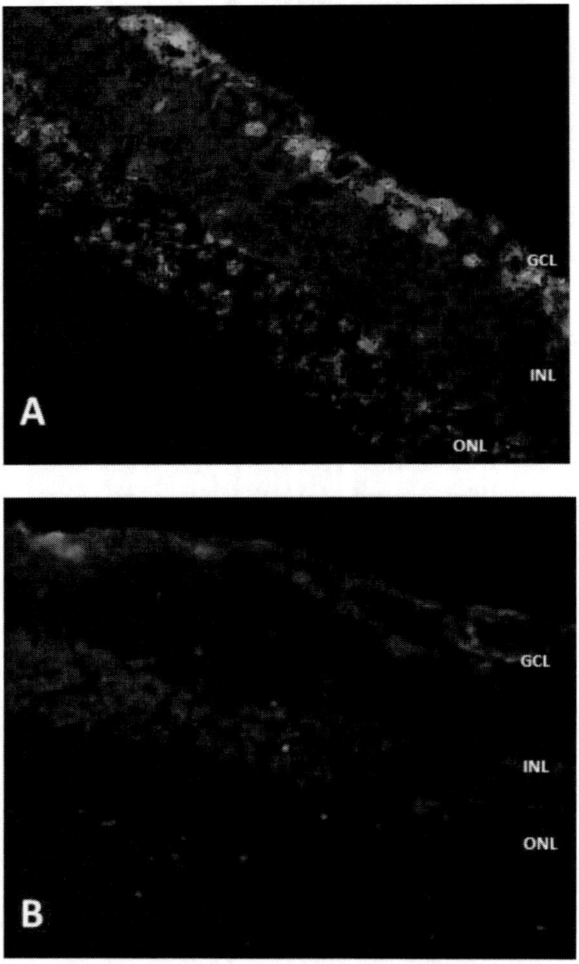

Figure 4. Rat retinas immunostained with iNOS antibodies 7 days after MTC injection without (A), or with (B) oral forskolin treatment. *GCL = ganglion cell layer; INL = inner nuclear layer; ONL = outer nuclear layer.*

Forskolin Modulates Caspase-3 Overexpression

Caspase 3 is the effector protein of apoptosis. Western blotting was carried out with protein extracts obtained from control, forskolin treated and untreated animals (Figure 5A). Quantitative analysis of the specific band was done by scanning the image, and the data normalized on the housekeeping protein actin are reported in the bar plot at the bottom (Figure 5 B). The ischemic damage induced by MTC injection resulted in a strong increase of caspase 3 (3.5 times with respect to the control), and forskolin supplementation in the diet reduced this increase to only a doubling.

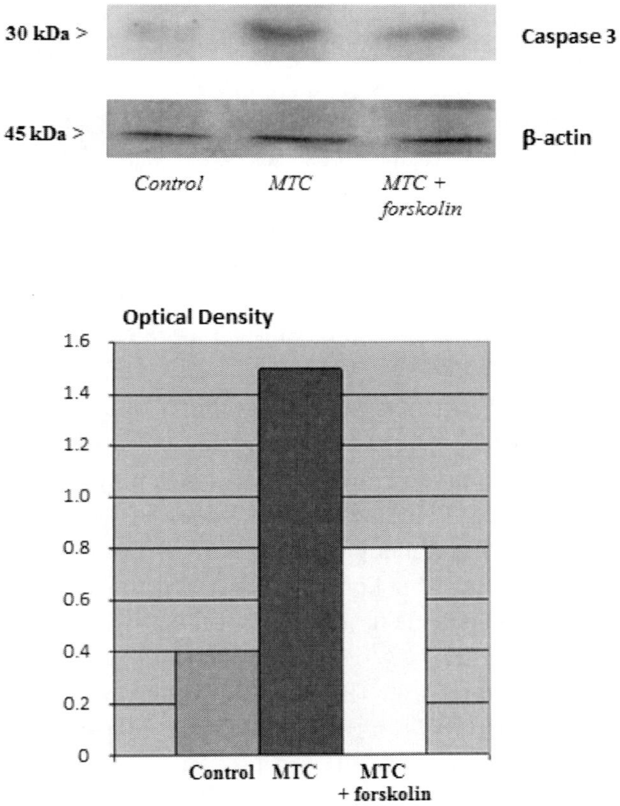

Figure 5. A representative western immuno-blot analysis of caspase 3 and actin extracted from retinas of untreated control animals, or animals 7 days after MTC injection without, or with oral forskolin treatment. B. Quantitative analysis of the western immuno-blot. Relative optical densities of caspase 3 bands normalized to actin values are reported in the histogram.

DISCUSSION

We have shown in this paper that forskolin administration to rats via the oral route is able to protect GCL neurons from ischemic damage, thus mimicking what could happen in hypertensive glaucoma. MTC impairment of aqueous humor outflow resulted in a two wave dramatic increase of the IOP during the first 3 h, which then stabilized at values higher than normal for the next 5 days. The ischemic damage following this treatment resulted in an enhanced expression of iNOS and a visible increase of free radicals (NADPH diaphorase assay: data not shown), which in turn induced caspase 3 synthesis, finally triggering apoptotic cell death of GCL neurons. Feeding the animals a diet enriched with forskolin could not prevent the initial peaks of IOP and the further acute ischemic damage, but resulted in a stabilization of the IOP at values that were somewhat lower than those attained without forskolin supplementation. Indeed, forskolin is known to be able to lower IOP after either topic administration as eye drops [38-39], or – to a lower extent – after oral administration as a human food supplement [40-42]. This activity of forskolin, especially after oral treatment, has a double relevance. First, it helps the hypotonizing effect of antiglaucoma eye drops and synergizes with almost all the commercially available antiglaucoma drugs [40-41]; second, it is a visible marker of the presence of forskolin within the eye, where it can also exert its neuroprotective activity.

In fact, forskolin, besides its facilitating effects on IOP control, has also shown several properties suggesting a possible role in neuroprotection. Peripheral nerve regeneration *in vivo* [30] and survival of rat RGCs in culture is significantly improved by the presence of forskolin, which allows the cells to respond to the growth promoting activity of the neurotrophins BDNF and CNTF [43]. Along this line, forskolin is known to stimulate the expression of BDNF in astrocytes and endothelial cells [44-45]. Furthermore, it promotes the translocation of the BDNF receptor TrkB to the RGC surface, thus making it available for ligand binding [46]. This may activate a survival paracrine circuit between these elements at the level of the retina. In fact, cAMP elevation following forskolin treatment enhances TrkB activation (phosphorylation) at low ligand doses (BDNF), and is still required to maintain its activation at higher ligand doses [47]. In a cat model of axonal regeneration after optic nerve transection, intravitreal injection of neurotrophins significantly improved survival of β ganglion cells only if forskolin was co-injected [48], indicating that also *in vivo* the action of cAMP is required to allow the functioning of the neurotrophin pathway.

Furthermore, systemic injection of forskolin in the rabbit resulted in a 43% increase of blood flow to the brain, despite a slight decrease in mean arterial pressure [49]. Adenyl-cyclase activity in the choroidal capillary endothelium was potently stimulated by forskolin, which also induced a vascular relaxing effect of the retinal capillary endothelium [50]. Such vascular activity of forskolin could also exert a neuroprotective effect on RGCs [51], albeit indirect.

Taken together, these results strongly suggest a neuroprotective activity of forskolin, which may be exerted at two levels: the first level involves indirect neuroprotection through an activity on the IOP and the blood flow, which might be responsible in our model system for decreased damage to the retina resulting in a lower production of iNOS and free radicals. The second level may involve direct neuroprotection, through the stimulation of the paracrine neurotrophin circuit based on BDNF and the cognate receptor TrkB, resulting in improved survival of RGCs and astrocytes and decreased activation of the apoptotic pathway. Such neuroprotective activity might also work in human glaucoma, as suggested by data recently published [52], in which POAG patients were treated with a food supplement containing forskolin and rutin, and showed a small but significant decrease of IOP and a significant improvement of the electric signaling (PERG) of RGCs.

More clinical studies are currently underway to show the neuroprotective activity of forskolin in association with other agents such as homotaurine and carnosine, and will be the subject of future publications.

ACKNOWLEDGMENTS

We thank Dr. Antony Bridgewood for the English proofreading of the manuscript.

AUTHOR DISCLOSURE STATEMENTS

N. Pescosolido, G. Scarsella: no competing financial interests exist

D. Rusciano is an employee of Sooft Italia Spa, a Company that produces a food supplement containing forskolin.

References

[1] Kwon, Y.H. Fingert, J.H. Kuehn, M.H. Alward, W.L. Primary open-angle glaucoma. *N. Engl. J. Med.* 2009; 360:1113-24.

[2] West, S.K. Looking forward to 20/20: a focus on the epidemiology of eye diseases. *Epidemiol. Rev. 2000*; 22:64-70.

[3] Friedman, D.S. Wilson, M.R. Liebmann, J.M. Fechtner, R.D. Weinreb, R.N. An evidence-based assessment of risk factors for the progression of ocular hypertension and glaucoma. *Am. J. Ophthalmol Rev.* 2004; 138:19–31.

[4] Morgan, J.E. Optic nerve head structure in glaucoma: astrocytes as mediators of axonal damage. *Eye.* 2000; 14:437–444.

[5] Ji, J. Chang, P. Pennesi, M.E. Yang , Z. Zhang , J. Li, D. Wu, S.M. Gross, R.L. Effects of elevated intraocular pressure on mouse retinal ganglion cells. *Vision Res.* 2005; 45:169–179.

[6] Calandrella, N. Scarsella, G. Pescosolido, N. Risuleo, G. Degenerative and apoptotic events at retinal and optic nerve level after experimental induction of ocular hypertension. *Mol. Cell Biochem.* 2007; 301:155–163.

[7] Leskea, M.C. Heijl, A. Hyman, L. Bengtsson, B. Komaroff, E. Factors for progression and glaucoma treatment: the Early Manifest Glaucoma Trial. *Curr. Opin. Ophthalmol.* 2004; 15:102-6.

[8] Miglior, S. Zeyen, T. Pfeiffer, N. Cunha-Vaz, J. Torri, V. Adamsons, I. European Glaucoma Prevention Study (EGPS) Group. Results of the European Glaucoma Prevention Study. *Ophthalmology.* 2005; 112:366-75.

[9] Coleman, A.L. Miglior, S. Risk factors for glaucoma onset and progression. *Surv Ophthalmol.* 2008; 53:S3-S10.

[10] Grieshaber, M.C. Flammer, J. Is the medication used to achieve the target intraocular pressure in glaucoma therapy of relevance? - An exemplary analysis on the basis of two beta-blockers. *Prog Retin Eye Res.* 2010; 29:79-93.

[11] Turaçli, M.E. Ozden, R.G. Gürses, M.A. The effect of betaxolol on ocular blood flow and visual fields in patients with normotension glaucoma. *Eur. J. Ophthalmol.* 1998; 8:62-6.

[12] Cheon, E.W, Park, C.H. Kang, S.S. Cho, G.J. Yoo, J.M. Song, J.K. Choi, W.S. Nitric oxide synthase expression in the transient ischemic rat retina: neuroprotection of betaxolol. *Neurosci Lett.* 2002; 330:265-9.

[13] Wood, J.P. DeSantis, L. Chao, H.M. Osborne, N.N. Topically applied betaxolol attenuates ischaemia-induced effects to the rat retina and stimulates BDNF mRNA. *Exp. Eye Res*. 2001; 72:79-86.

[14] Krupin, T. Liebmann, J.M. Greenfield, D.S. Ritch, R. Gardiner, S. Low-Pressure Glaucoma Study Group. A randomized trial of brimonidine versus timolol in preserving visual function: results from the Low-Pressure Glaucoma Treatment Study. *Am. J. Ophthalmol.* 2011; 151:671-81.

[15] De Souza, N.J. Dohadwalla, A.N. Reden, J. Forskolin: A labdane diterpenoid with antihypertensive, positive inotropic, platelet aggregation inhibitory and adenylate cyclase activating properties. *Med. Res Rev* 1983; 3:201-19.

[16] Valdes, L.J. Mislankar, S.G. Paul, A.G. Coleus Barbatus, C. Forskohlii Lamiaceae and the potential new drug Forskolin Coleonol. *Econ Bot.* 1987; 44:474-83.

[17] Ammon, H.P. Muller, A.B. Forskolin: From an ayurvedic remedy to a modern agent. *Planta Med.* 1985; 46:473-7.

[18] Ammon, H.P. Kemper, F.H. Ayurveda: 3000 years of Indian traditional medicine. *Med Welt.* 1982; 33:148-53.

[19] Seamon, K.B. Daly, J.W. Forskolin: A unic diterpene activator of cyclic AMP generating systems. *J. Cyclic Nucleotide Res*. 1981; 7:220-1.

[20] Barber, R. Goka, T.J. Adenylate cyclase activity as a function of forskolin concentration. *J. Cyclic Nucleotide Protein Phosphor. Res.* 1985; 10:23-9.

[21] Rojas, F.J. Bruzzone, M.E. Regulation of cyclic adenosine monophosphate synthesis in human ejaculated spermatozoa. I. Experimental conditions to quantitate membrane-bound adenylyl cyclase activity. *Hum Reprod.* 1992; 7:1126-30.

[22] Zhang, X. Wang, N. Schroeder, A. Erickson, K.A. Expression of adenylate cyclase subtypes II and IV in the human outflow pathway. *Invest Ophthalmol Vis Sci*. 2000; 41:998-1005.

[23] Busch, M.J. Kobayashi, K. Hoyng, P.F. Mittag, T.W. Adenylyl cyclase in human and bovine trabecular meshwork. *Invest Ophthalmol Vis Sci.* 1993; 34:3028-34.

[24] Caprioli, J. Sears, M. Bausher, L. Gregory, D. Mead, A. Forskolin lowers intraocular pressure by reducing aqueous inflow. *Invest Ophthalmol. Vis. Sci*. 1984; 25:268-77.

[25] Caprioli, J. Sears, M. Forskolin lowers intraocular pressure in rabbits, monkeys, and man. *Lancet*. 1983; 1:958-60.

[26] Shen, X. Koga, T. Park, B.C. SundarRaj, N. Yue, B.Y. Rho GTPase and cAMP/protein kinase A signaling mediates myocilin-induced alterations in cultured human trabecular meshwork cells. *J. Biol. Chem.* 2008; 283:603-12.
[27] Ramachandran, C. Satpathy, M. Mehta, D. Srinivas, S.P. Forskolin induces myosin light chain dephosphorylation in bovine trabecular meshwork cells. *Curr Eye Res.* 2008; 33:169-76.
[28] Yu, M. Chen, X. Wang, N. Cai, S. Li, N. Qiu, J. Brandt, C.R. Kaufman, P.L. Liu, X. H-1152 effects on intraocular pressure and trabecular meshwork morphology of rat eyes. *J. Ocul Pharmacol Ther.* 2008; 24:373-9.
[29] Honjo, M. Inatani, M. Kido, N. Sawamura, T. Yue, B.Y. Honda, Y. Tanihara, H. Effects of protein kinase inhibitor, HA1077, on intraocular pressure and outflow facility in rabbit eyes. *Arch. Ophthalmol.* 2001; 119:1171-8.
[30] Kilmer, S.L. Carlsen, R.C. Forskolin activation of adenylate cyclase in vivo stimulates nerve regeneration. *Nature.* 1984; 307:455-7.
[31] Zhu, M.D. Cai, F.Y. Development of experimental chronic intraocular hypertension in the rabbit. *Aust N Z J Ophthalmol.* 1992; 20:225-34.
[32] Irwin, S. Comprehensive observational assessment: Ia. A systematic, quantitative procedure for assessing the behavioral and physiologic state of the mouse. *Psychopharmacologia.* 1968; 13:222-257.
[33] Scarsella, G. Nebbioso, M. Stefanini, S. Librando, A. Pescosolido, N. Degenerative effects in rat eyes after experimental ocular hypertension. *Eur J Histochem.* 2012; 56: e42.
[34] Calandrella N, Scarsella G, Pescosolido N, Risuleo G. Degenerative and apoptotic events at retinal and optic nerve level after experimental induction of ocular hypertension. *Mol. Cell Biochem.* 2007; 301: 155-63.
[35] Nebbioso M, Scarsella G, Tafani M, Pescosolido N. Mechanisms of ocular neuroprotection by antioxidant molecules in animal models. *J. Biol. Regul Homeost Agents.* 2013; 27:197-209.
[36] Laemmli, U.K. Cleavage of structural proteins during the assembly of the head of bacteriophage T4. *Nature.* 1970; 227:680-5.
[37] Shah AM. Inducible nitric oxide synthase and cardiovascular disease. *Cardiovasc Res.* 2000; 45:148-55.
[38] Caprioli, J. Sears, M. The adenylate cyclase receptor complex and aqueous humor formation. *Yale J. Biol Med.* 1984; 57:283-300.

[39] Gupta, S. Samanta, M.K. Design and evaluation of thermoreversible in situ gelling system of forskolin for the treatment of glaucoma. *Pharm Dev Technol.* 2010; 15:386-93.

[40] Pescosolido, N. Librando, A. Oral administration of an association of forskolin, rutin and vitamins B1 and B2 potentiates the hypotonising effects of pharmacological treatments in POAG patients. *Clin. Ter.* 2010; 161:81-5.

[41] Vetrugno, M. Uva, M.G. Russo, V, Iester, M. Ciancaglini, M. Brusini, P. Centofanti, M. Rossetti, L.M. Oral administration of forskolin and rutin contributes to intraocular pressure control in primary open angle glaucoma patients under maximum tolerated medical therapy. *J. Ocul Pharmacol Ther.* 2012; 28:536-41.

[42] Nebbioso, M. Belcaro, G. Librando, A. Rusciano, D. Steigerwalt, R.D. Jr. Pescosolido, N. Forskolin and rutin prevent intraocular pressure spikes after Nd:YAG laser iridotomy. *Panminerva Med.* 2012; 54:77-82.

[43] Meyer-Franke, A. Kaplan, M.R. Pfrieger, F.W. Barres, B.A. Characterization of the signaling interactions that promote the survival and growth of developing retinal ganglion cells in culture. *Neuron.* 1995; 15:805-19.

[44] Juric, D.M. Loncar, D. Carman-Krzan, M. Noradrenergic stimulation of BDNF synthesis in astrocytes: mediation via alpha1- and beta1/beta2-adrenergic receptors. *Neurochem. Int.* 2008; 52:297-306.

[45] Nakahashi, T. Fujimura, H. Altar, C.A. Li, J. Kambayashi, J. Tandon, N.N. Sun, B. Vascular endothelial cells synthesize and secrete brain-derived neurotrophic factor. *FEBS Lett.* 2000; 470:113-7.

[46] Meyer-Franke, A. Wilkinson, G.A. Kruttgen, A. Hu, M. Munro, E. Hanson, M.G.Jr. Reichardt, L.F. Barres, B.A. Depolarization and cAMP elevation rapidly recruit TrkB to the plasma membrane of CNS neurons. *Neuron.* 1998; 21:681-93.

[47] Ji, Y. Pang, P.T. Feng, L. Lu, B. Cyclic AMP controls BDNF-induced TrkB phosphorylation and dendritic spine formation in mature hippocampal neurons. *Nat. Neurosci.* 2005; 8:164-72.

[48] Watanabe, M. Fukuda, Y. Survival and axonal regeneration of retinal ganglion cells in adult cats. *Prog. Retin Eye Res.* 2002; 21:529-53.

[49] Wysham, D.G. Brotherton, A.F. Heistad, D.D. Effects of forskolin on cerebral blood flow: implications for a role of adenylate cyclase. *Stroke.* 1986; 17:1299-303.

[50] Haefliger, I.O. Chen, Q. Anderson, D.R. Effect of oxygen on relaxation of retinal pericytes by sodium nitroprusside. *Graefes Arch. Clin. Exp Ophthalmol.* 1997; 235:388-92.
[51] Chiou, G.C. Xu, X.R. Effects of some natural flavonoids on retinal function recovery after ischemic insult in the rat. *J. Ocul Pharmacol Ther.* 2004; 20:107-13.
[52] Sisto, D., Lavermicocca, N., Errico, D. and Rusciano, D. Oral administration of forskolin and rutin contributes to reduce intraocular pressure and improves PERG (pattern electroretinogram) amplitude in glaucomatous patients. *JSM Biotechnol Bioeng.* 2013; 2: 1036.

Reviewed by:

Dr. Claudio Bucolo, PhD, Department of Clinical and Molecular Biomedicine, Section of Pharmacology and Biochemistry, Medical School, University of Catania, Catania, Italy. bucocla@unict.it

Dr. Massimo Dal Monte, PhD, Department of Biology, University of Pisa, Via San Zeno, 31, 56127, Pisa, Italy. massimo.dalmonte@unipi.it

Dr. Rossella Russo, PhD, Department of Pharmacy, Health and Nutritional Sciences, University of Calabria, Arcavacata di Rende, Italy. rossella.russo@unical.it

In: Forskolin
Editor: Marty H. Walker
ISBN: 978-1-63463-918-7

Chapter 3

FORSKOLIN EMBRYOTOXICITY IN INITIAL STAGES OF THE EMBRYONIC DEVELOPMENT IN CHICK

Lucia de Fatima Sobral Sampaio[1*],
Renato Correa Nogueira[1]
and Maria Auxiliadora Pantoja Ferreira[2]
[1]Laboratory of Biochemistry of the Central Nervous System Development, Biological Sciences Institute, Federal University of Pará, Belém, PA, Brazil
[2]Laboratory of Immunohistochemistry and Biology of Development, Biological Sciences Institute, Federal University of Pará, Belém, PA, Brazil

ABSTRACT

Since 1971, forskolin has been widely used in research because it activates the ATP pyrophosphate-lyase (cyclizing) enzyme system, EC 4.6.1.1 (adenylate cyclase, AC), resulting in increased cAMP levels. Recently, this terpene has been used as a natural supplement to treat arterial hypertension and asthma through its ability to relax blood vessels. However, animal models have suggested that forskolin may have potential embryotoxicity and teratogenicity in human embryos. Studies

[*] Corresponding author: mail to lsampaio@ufpa.br.

show that forskolin is dangerous to the cardiovascular system in developing chick embryos at Hamburger-Hamilton stage 24 (HH24), a stage in which the developing cardiovascular system is modulated by catecholamines. This chapter studies forskolin-induced morphological changes in the cardiovascular system, even when applied in embryos at the HH12 stage, which is characterized by the absence of the catecholaminergic machinery. Eggs containing chick embryos that were incubated for 48 h (HH12-13) were grouped into basal, control and test groups. Embryos were assayed *in ovo* by injection of 10 µl of forskolin solutions (1.07 x 10^{-12} mol/egg; 4.14 x 10^{-12} mol/egg; 8.29 x 10^{-12} mol/egg; 15.58 x 10^{-12} mol/egg; 33.16 x 10^{-12} mol/egg and 66.33 x 10^{-12} mol/egg) in the air camera of the yolk sac. The basal group did not receive an injection, while the control group was injected with 10 µl of distilled water. No lethality was observed at HH18, when the morphology of the area vasculosa (AV) and the whole embryo was observed. In eggs from the test group, the phenotype of both the AV and the embryo were disrupted depending on the amount of forskolin injected. In contrast, normal cardiovascular development was observed in the AV and in the whole embryos from the basal and control groups.

In conclusion, forskolin is potentially toxic for extraembryonic vascular tissues and embryonic cardiovascular system development, even at stages where this system is resistant to catecholamines. These results suggest that forskolin is contraindicated for women who are planning a pregnancy.

1. INTRODUCTION

1.1. Forskolin and the Adenylate Cyclase Enzyme

Forskolin is a labdane diterpene obtained from *Coleus forskohlii*. It has been widely used in research because it activates the ATP pyrophosphate-lyase (cyclizing), EC 4.6.1.1 (adenylate cyclase, AC), enzyme system [1] by binding to this enzyme [2, 3] and stabilizing its catalytic subunit [4]. In contrast, essential oils rich in the monoterpene linalool inhibit AC, without apparent effects on active site stability [5].

AC is an integral membrane protein that presents its catalytic subunit on the cytosolic side of the membrane [6, 7] and is present in both eukaryotic and prokaryotic cells [8, 9]. ATP is the AC substrate for cAMP synthesis [10, 11]. This second-messenger has many functions, including development [12, 13], metabolism [14], muscular tonus control [15] and other functions [16, 17].

Therefore, AC activity depends on the extracellular demand, which is signaled by neurotransmitters [18] and hormones [19] that bind to seven transmembrane domain receptors coupled to G proteins (GPCRs), specifically Gi or Gs proteins. These proteins negatively (Gi) and positively (Gs) modulate the AC enzyme activity [20, 21]. AC activity is also modulated by neurotransmitters and hormones that signal by modulating cytosolic calcium waves and/or the activity of the calcium-binding protein calmodulin [22]. Accordingly, a myriad of cellular functions are assessed using forskolin.

The ability of forskolin to increase cAMP levels promotes blood vessel relaxation [23, 24, 25, 26] and bronchodilation [27]. Therefore, direct stimulation of AC is the basis of forskolin use as a natural supplement to treat arterial hypertension [28] and asthma [29]. However, in accord with the forskolin MSDS (Material Safety Data Sheet, last Updated: 06/09/2012), there is no information available regarding the potential teratogenicity and embryotoxicity of forskolin in humans.

1.2. Forskolin Embryotoxicity in Chick Embryos

The chick embryo is an established model for screening teratogenicity because it is more susceptive to teratogens than mammalian species, which makes it a good model to perform preclinical assays prior to testing drug candidates in mammals [30]. Hamburger and Hamilton (HH) created the most used series of normal stages of chick embryo development. It comprises 46 stages, including newly hatched chicks at 21 days [31]. Normal chick embryonic development occurs as a function of the health of both the extraembryonic membranes and embryonic blood vessels.

The extraembryonic membranes comprise the yolk sac that contain the nutritive material, the amnion that functions as a protective cushion that permits the embryo to exercise, and the chorion that contain both of these membranes. The other membrane present from the beginning of development is the allantois, which functions both as the respiratory organ and receives the excretions of the embryonic kidneys; it also absorbs albumen (a protein surge) and calcium from the shell. After the first 4 days of incubation, the allantois membrane progressively fuses with the mesodermal layer of the chorion, until the chorioallantoic membrane (CAM) is completely formed, up to day 19 [32]. The CAM begins to make contact with the egg shell membrane on day 6, until the egg content is completely enveloped on day 12 [32]. The embryonic blood vessels can be divided into the viteline vessels that carry nutritive material for development, and the allantois vessels that carry waste material from the embryo and are responsible for respiration. At up to 6 days of incubation, the viteline vessels of the area vasculosa (AV) are the respiratory organ [33]. Afterward, they are replaced by the vessels of the CAM, which is the avian homologue of the mammalian placenta [32, 33]. At initial developmental stages, CAM vessels are unresponsive to contraction agents [34]. However, an interesting study showed that forskolin relaxes CAM arteries in chick embryos regardless of age or the presence of pre-contraction agents such as acetylcholine [35], but this study did not identify whether this also occurs at the AV, the main respiratory organ, before the start of CAM formation [36]. This information should be important because could be able to predict forskolin embryotoxicity in the initial stages of mammalian species development, when fetoplacental circulation is still in process. In fact, adequate blood supply to the fetus depends on the vasomotor tone in the vessels of the fetoplacental circulation [37].

The circulatory system is the first system to develop in chick. The heart becomes autonomous at 33-45 h of incubation (HH10-11), when the primary heart tube is formed, and the transformation of the straight heart tube into the c shaped heart tube (dextral-looping phase) begins. Cardiac looping occurs in two time frames, the first is the early phase of the cardiac looping at 29 h - 4 days (HH9-24), and the second is the late phase of cardiac septation at 4-8 days (HH24-34). Three-day-old chick embryos (HH12 and HH13) have a tubular heart structure with one atrium and one ventricle, and the embryonic circulation begins at HH13 [38].

Both the CAM and the chick heart are more resistant to exogenous neurotransmitters, such as norepinephrine, epinephrine, dopamine, and to the β-blockers propranolol and atenolol in early embryonic stages than in later stages of prenatal development [39, 40, 41]. This most likely occurs because these compounds function to modulate AC by binding to GPCRs. Developmental expression profiles of the α–subunit of the Gs and Gi proteins are characterized by lower levels during early heart development, and higher levels between embryonic days 4 to 8 that remaining unchanged up to embryonic day 18. In contrast, AC expression and forskolin sensitivity is the same during this time frame, where the tissues can be stimulated by forskolin. Only the total amount of AC5, the principal cardiac AC isoform, decreases between embryonic days 12 and 18, remaining constant from embryonic day 18 to hatching, which contrasts with the increase in the levels of the Gi and Gs proteins [41]. Remarkably, the AC activity is measurable beginning at 24 h of incubation in homogenates of whole chick embryos, increasing up to embryonic day 3 and decreasing slightly prior to embryonic day 10 before remaining constant up to embryonic day 20 [42]. The developmental profile of the cAMP levels measured in total developing heart homogenates shows higher cAMP levels up to day 4, decreasing sharply at day 5, and gradually decreasing to a plateau level at day 16 [43]. Therefore, the cAMP levels are the inverse of the Gs and Gi protein profiles [41]. These results suggest that the cardiac isoform of adenylate cyclase, AC5 [44], is under negative modulation at the time in which cardiac septation [38] is occurring.

The cardiotoxic effects of forskolin application (10^{-9} to 10^{-7} mol/egg) to the extraembryonic membranes of eggs that were incubated for 4 days (HH24) were observed in embryos at 14 days of incubation (HH40). Doses less than 10^{-8} mol egg/did not affect the survival rate. The rate of cardiac malformations caused by 10^{-8} to 10^{-7} mol/egg of forskolin was concentration-dependent and characterized by persistent defects of the left fourth aortic arch and ventricular septum [45]. Similar forskolin-dependent cardiotoxic effects were further analyzed in this model by the additional application of IBMX and caffeine, methylxanthines that function to increase cAMP levels. Forskolin potentiated the effect of the methylxanthines at concentrations around their EC_{50}, confirming that the cardiotoxic effects of the methylxanthines and forskolin itself were mediated by the increased cAMP levels [46].

As forskolin functions mainly by directly activating the adenylate cyclase enzyme [3], the AV and the whole embryo may be sensitive to forskolin, even in early developmental stages, when the coupling between transmitters and effectors has not developed. In this chapter, forskolin embryotoxicity was evaluated in 3 day old chick embryos at HH18 that had been exposed to forskolin beginning at HH12.

2. Materials and Methods

2.1. Materials

Forskolin was purchased from Tocris Cookson Limited (UK).

2.2. Animals

Fertile chicken eggs (112) were provided from a local hatchery. They were placed vertically in an automatic incubator, with humid atmosphere, at

37.78 °C (Dove Factories, Vinhedo, SP, Brazil). The first day of the incubation was counted as “day 0”. The protocol received the approved of the Ethics Committee in Research with Experimental Animals of the Federal University of Pará (CEPAE-UFPA: 229-14).

2.3. Assay of the Forskolin Embryotoxicity in the Chick Embryo (*In Ovo*)

2.3.1. Preparation of the Forskolin

Forskolin was dissolved with 50% absolute alcohol to a concentration of 7×10^{-3} M. This high concentration forskolin solution was diluted by 50% with distilled water, and, thereafter, diluted again by 50%, to create a complete battery of forskolin solutions at six concentrations: 0.21×10^{-3} M; 0.42×10^{-3} M; 0.85×10^{-3} M; 1.7×10^{-3} M; 3.5×10^{-3} and 7×10^{-3} M.

2.3.2. Embryotoxicity Assay

The embryos were staged according with Hamburger and Hamilton staging series (HH) [31]. Fertile chicken eggs (112) were distributed in 3 groups: basal (n=14), control (n=14) and forskolin-treated (n=14 embryos for each concentration). A total of the 5 experiments were performed.

The total volume of the egg at day 0 is approximately 65 ml. All eggs were incubated in the vertical position with the air sac located at the top of the egg for 48 h, at which time the embryos are developing to HH12. At room temperature (20 °C), a small hole was created above the air camera of the yolk sac to inoculate the eggs with 10 μl of each forskolin solution. The amount of forskolin inoculated was 1.07×10^{-12} mol/egg, 4.14×10^{-12} mol/egg, 8.29×10^{-12} mol/egg, 15.58×10^{-12} mol/egg, 33.16×10^{-12} mol/egg and 66.33×10^{-12} mol/egg. Control eggs were inoculated with distilled water (10 μl). The small hole in the egg was closed with a microporous tape. Next, the eggs were incubated for 18 h to HH18. At this stage, basal, control and forskolin-treated eggs were opened at the air sac region, and the vessels of the area vasculosa (AV) were manually analyzed and photographed with a common digital camera. The embryos were excised and washed in a PBS solution. Then, they were maintained at 4 °C in a PBS solution, in which the embryos were imaged and analyzed with an optical microscope, (Bioval L-1000B) coupled to a digital camera (Nikon Coolpix 2300).

3. RESULTS

3.1. Forskolin Disrupts the Morphology of the Area Vasculosa (AV)

The morphology of the AV vasculature from chicken eggs of each experimental group was manually observed 18 h after forskolin treatment. No differences were observed in the AV morphology between the basal and control groups; both groups displayed right and left viteline vessels with abundant branches around the embryos (Figure 1a and b). However, this was not observed with forskolin treatment. In embryos subjected to forskolin at doses equal to or higher than 1.07 x 10^{-12} mol/egg (Figure 1c, d, e, f, g, h), a gradual increase in the caliber of the vessels was observed, with the largest expansion observed in the caliber of the main trunk vessels (Figure 1c, d, e and f). Forskolin applications at 33.16 x 10^{-12} mol/egg and above triggered an apparent reduction in the diameter of both the left and right main vessels and in the number of branches around the embryo (Figure 1 g and h). Thus, chicken eggs containing embryos at HH12 that were exposed to forskolin for 18 h exhibited a dose-dependent disturbance in the morphology of the area vasculosa at HH18.

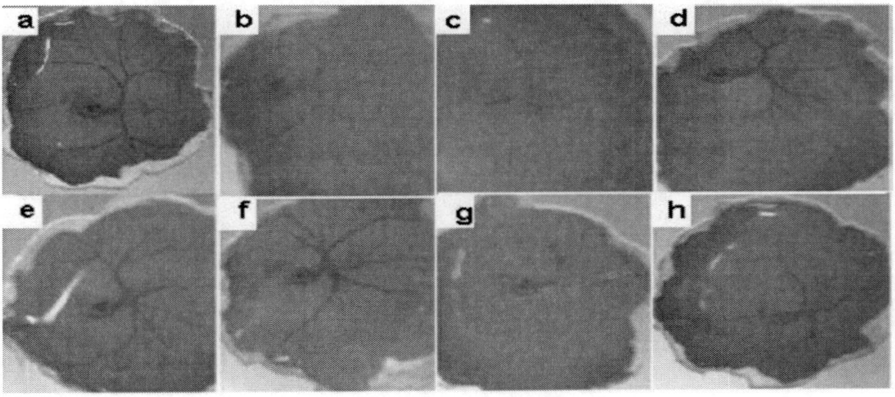

Figure 1. Dose-dependent disturbance in the phenotype of the area vasculosa in forskolin-treated (at HH12-13 or 48 h of incubation) fertile chicken eggs incubated by 66 h (HH18) that received forskolin at 48 h of the incubation (HH12-13). Basal, a. Control (10 μl of distillated water), b. Forskolin 1.07 x 10^{-12} mol/egg, c; 4.14 x 10^{-12} mol/egg, d; 8.29 x 10^{-12} mol/egg, e; 15.58 x 10^{-12} mol/egg, f; 33.16 x 10^{-12} mol/egg, g and 66.33 x 10^{-12} mol/egg, h. Each image is a representative result from 14 experiments.

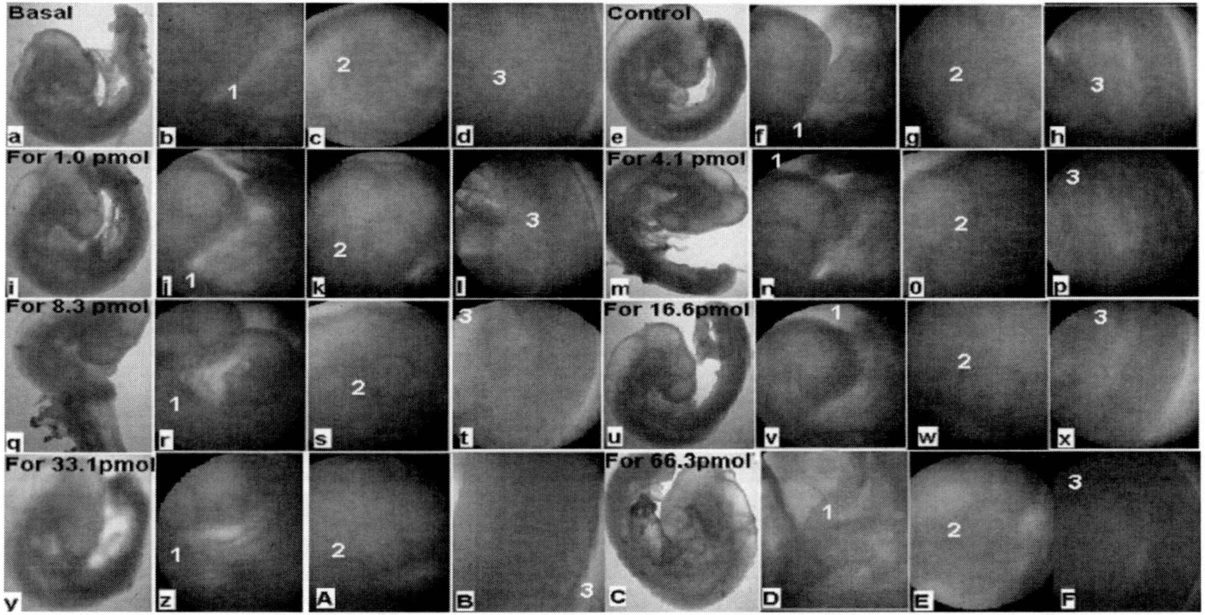

Figure 2. Forskolin-mediated embryotoxicity in freshly dissected HH18 chick embryos immersed in a PBS solution. Antero-lateral views of a representative embryo from each group showing the heart (1), eye cup (2) and embryonic trunk (3). Compared with embryos from the basal group (a, b, c, d), the morphology of embryos from the control group (e, f, g, h) and the 1.07×10^{-12} mol/egg forskolin-treated group (i, j, k, l) were similar. In the 4.14×10^{-12} mol/egg forskolin-treated group (m, n, o, p) and higher dose groups (q, r, s, t, u, v, w, x, y, z, A, B, C, D, E, F), a dose-dependent alteration in the morphology of the developing cardiovascular system and eye cup was observed. The magnification was 25x, except for whole chick embryos (a, e, i, m, q, u, A, E) which was 10x. Each image is representative of the 14 embryos in each group.

3.2. Forskolin Embryotoxicity in Chick Embryos at HH18

Forskolin application to the air camera of the yolk sac containing chick embryos at HH12 caused morphological disturbances in the chick embryos at HH18 (Figure 2). The morphology of the embryos from the basal group was in accord with the Hamburger & Hamilton standard [31]. In chick embryos treated with 1.07 x 10^{-12} mol/egg of the forskolin for 18 h, the areas of the atrium and ventricles (Figure 2 j) and the dorsal aortas (Figure 2 l) displayed a normal shape and size, similar to embryos from basal (Figure 2 b and d) and control groups (Figure 2 f and h). However, the heart of embryos treated with forskolin at doses of 4.14 x 10^{-12} mol/egg (Figure 2 n and p) and 8.29 x 10^{-12} mol/egg (Figure 2 r and t) exhibited a slight enlargement of the ventricular and atrial cavities, with a discrete increase in the heart wall thickness. In these animals, the diameter of the dorsal aorta was enlarged, with an apparent increase in blood flow. At a forskolin dose of 16.29 x 10^{-12} mol/egg, a sharp increase in both cavities and the wall thickness of the atrium and ventricle (Figure 2 v, z and D) were observed and were associated with blood retention, especially in the atrial cavity (Figure 2 z and D). In the dorsal region of the trunk, the presence of dilated dorsal aortas and intersomitic arteries were observed (Figure 2 p, t, x, B and F). The optical chalice of all forskolin-treated embryos was formed, but exhibited dose-dependent levels of hemorrhage and edema. These results are summarized in Table 1. No lethality was observed in embryos from forskolin-treated groups observed at HH18.

Table 1.

*Forskolin x!0^{-12}/egg	Heart with aberrant phenotype	Trunk/ cup optic with aberrant vascularization	**HH12/ HH18
None or *distilled water	-	-	14/14
1.07	-	-	14/14
4.14	+/-	+/-	14/14
8.29	+	+/-	14/14
16.58	++	+	14/14
33.16	+++	++	14/14
66.33	+++	+++	14/14

*Volume applied 10 μl.

** Ratio of the number of embryos alive at time of the experiment and at the time of the eggs opening.

4. Discussion

During the third day of incubation, the AV is the main place of the gas exchange for the chick embryo. The cardiac loop is completed, with the transformation of the c-shaped heart loop and s-shaped heart loop [38]. The inoculation of forskolin in the air camera of the yolk sac caused a dose-dependent aberrant phenotype in the vessels of the area vasculosa that was characterized by the enlargement and reduced branching of the main vessels. In the embryonic vasculature and heart, aberrant vessel morphology and edema were observed. These results are in accord with a study showing that whole Xenopus embryos at Nieuwkoop-Faber stage 31 (NF31) displayed edema, defective angiogenesis, impaired intersomitic vessels and a hypoplastic viteline vein network when incubated in culture medium supplemented with forskolin (20×10^{-6} M) from NF29-30 (4 days). Periocular, pericardial, ventral, and pronephric edema are also observed in the Xenopus embryos [47] and in the chick embryos at HH18 shown here.

Other studies on forskolin teratogenicity [45, 46] were performed in chick embryos at the late phase of cardiac septation, which begins at 4 days of incubation (HH24) [38]. In those studies, forskolin was applied at 10^{-8} to 10^{-7} mol/egg on the CAM, inducing dose-dependent ventricular septal defects and persistence of the fourth aortic arch [45], likely by elevation of the cAMP levels [46]. At this stage, the catecholaminergic machinery is ready and the AC modulation occurs mainly by GPCRs [41]. It is not known if vasodilation and edema precede the cardiac teratogenic effects of forskolin applied at HH24, but it is highly plausible. Therefore, forskolin embryotoxicity is likely due to cAMP increases that cause edema by acting on vascular smooth muscle through increased blood flow [48].

Because forskolin has a lipophilic nature, the amount applied in the air camera of the yolk sac reaches both the AV and the embryo. Therefore, at HH12, the embryo receives the amount of forskolin that crosses the extraembryonic membranes and the amount that reaches the vessels of the AV. Thus, another point to be discussed is the relationship between the vascular dilation in the AV and the forskolin embryotoxicity observed in these stages. Vasodilation leads to embryonic hypotension and anoxia that causes cardiac malformations [49]. The amount of the forskolin applied that reaches the embryo was not estimated here, but, interestingly, HH18 embryos from the lowest dose forskolin-treated group (1.07×10^{-12} mol/egg) were devoid of any morphological alteration, even though the vessels of the AV exhibited a slightly disrupted morphology. However, the amount of forskolin that crossed the extraembryonic membranes had a role in the embryotoxicity observed in embryos from forskolin-treated groups.

CONCLUSION

The vital activity of AC, the primary forskolin target, is present from the formation of the vertebrate embryo. The positive modulation of this enzyme by forskolin is responsible for the embryotoxicity observed in developing chick embryos in this and other studies. Due to the similar function of the developing cardiovascular system among vertebrates, the present research indicates that pregnant women, or those who are planning pregnancy, need to be aware that forskolin is dangerous for the developing cardiovascular system.

ACKNOWLEDGMENTS

The undergraduate student, Renato Correa Nogueira, is a PIBIC/UFPA-AF fellow. This research was supported by grants from CNPq.

REFERENCES

[1] Alasbahi R.H.& Melzig, M. F. (2012). Forskolin and derivatives as tools for studying the role of cAMP. *Pharmazie.*, 67, 5-13.

[2] Seamon, K. B., Padgett, W., & Daly, J. W. (1981). Forskolin: unique diterpene activator of adenylate cyclase in membranes and in intact cells. *Proceedings of the National Academy of Sciences,* 78, 3363-3367.

[3] Seamon, K., & Daly, J. W. (1981). Activation of adenylate cyclase by the diterpene forskolin does not require the guanine nucleotide regulatory protein. *Journal of Biological Chemistry,* 256, 9799-9801.

[4] Green, D. A., & Clark, R. B. (1981). Direct evidence for the role of the coupling proteins in forskolin activation of adenylate cyclase. *Journal of cyclic nucleotide research, 8,* 337-346.

[5] Sampaio L. F. S., Maia J. G., de Parijós, A. M., de Souza, R. Z. & Barata, L. E. (2012). Linalool from rosewood (Aniba rosaeodora Ducke)

oil inhibits adenylate cyclase in the retina, contributing to understanding its biological activity. *Phytotheraphy Research,* 26, 73-77.

[6] Ross, E. M. & Gilman, A. G. (1977). Resolution of some components of adenylate cyclase necessary for catalytic activity. *Journal of Biological Chemistry,* 252, 6966-6969.

[7] Northup, J. K., Sternweis, P. C., Smigel, M. D., Schleifer, L. S., Ross, E. M. & Gilman, A. G. (1980). Purification of the regulatory component of adenylate cyclase. *Proceedings of the National Academy of Sciences, 77*, 6516-6520.

[8] Vauquelin, G., Geynet, P., Hanoune, J. & Strosberg, A. D. (1977). Isolation of adenylate cyclase-free, beta-adrenergic receptor from turkey erythrocyte membranes by affinity chromatography. *Proceedings of the National Academy of Sciences,* 74, 3710-3714.

[9] Wolff, J., Cook, G. H., Goldhammer, A. R. & Berkowitz, S. A. (1980). Calmodulin activates prokaryotic adenylate cyclase. *Proceedings of the National Academy of Sciences,* 77, 3841-3844.

[10] Yoram, S, Londos, C. & Rodbell, M. (1975). “A highly sensitive adenylate cyclase assay". *Analytical biochemistry, 58*, 541-548.

[11] Seamon, K. B. & Daly, J. W. (1980). Forskolin: a unique diterpene activator of cyclic AMP-generating systems. *Journal of cyclic nucleotide research,* 7, 201-224.

[12] Dunn, T. A. & Feller M. B. (2008). Imaging second messenger dynamics in developing neural circuits. *Developmental Neurobiology,* 68, 835-844.

[13] Sampaio, L. F. S. (2009). cAMP and Neurodevelopment. In: Benito Figueredo & Fidel Meléndez (Eds.), *Neuroscience Research Advances,* (edition: 1ed, .pp. 191-203). New York, NY. Nova Science Publishers Inc.

[14] Madsen, L. & Kristiansen, K. (2010). The importance of dietary modulation of cAMP and insulin signaling in adipose tissue and the development of obesity. *Annals of the New York Academy of Sciences.* 1190, 1-14.

[15] Berdeaux, R. & Stewart, R. (2012). cAMP signaling in skeletal muscle adaptation:hypertrophy, metabolism, and regeneration. *American Journal of Physiology Endocrinology and Metabolism,* 303, 1-17.

[16] Pace, U., Hanski, E., Salomon, Y., & Lancet, D. (1985). Odorant-sensitive adenylate cyclase may mediate olfactory reception. *Nature,* 316, 255-258.

[17] O'Neill, J. S, Maywood, E. S. & Hastings, M. H. (2013). Cellular mechanisms of circadian pacemaking: beyond transcriptional loops. in Akim Kramer & Martha Merrow (Eds.), *Circadian clocks,* 67-103. Berlin, Heidelberg, Springer.

[18] Sampaio, L.F. & Paes-de-Carvalho, R. (1998). Developmental regulation of group III metabotropic glutamate receptors modulating adenylate cyclase activity in the avian retina. *Neurochemistry International,* 33, 367-74.

[19] Ross, E. M. & Gilman, A. G. (1980). Biochemical properties of hormone-sensitive adenylate cyclase. *Annual Review of Biochemistry,* 49, 533-564.

[20] Limbird, L. E. (1981). Activation and attenuation of adenylate cyclase. The role of GTP-binding proteins as macromolecular messengers in receptor-cyclase coupling. *Biochemical Journal,* 195(1), 1.

[21] Gilman, A. G. (1984). G proteins and dual control of adenylate cyclase. *Cell,* 36, 577-579.

[22] Wang, H. & Storm, D. R. (2003). Calmodulin-regulated adenylyl cyclases: cross-talk and plasticity in the central nervous system. *Molecular pharmacology*, 63, 463-468.

[23] Harraz, O. F. & Welsh, D. G. (2013). Protein kinase A regulation of T-type Ca2+ channels in rat cerebral arterial smooth muscle. *Journal of Cell Sciences,* 126, 2944-2954.

[24] Zieba, B. J., Artamonov, M. V., Jin, L., Momotani, K., Ho, R., Franke, A. S., Neppl, R. L., Stevenson, A. S., Khromov, A. S., Chrzanowska-Wodnicka, M. & Somlyo, A. V. (2011). The cAMP-responsive Rap1 guanine nucleotide exchange factor, Epac, induces smooth muscle relaxation by down-regulation of RhoA activity. *The Journal of Biological Chemistry,* 286, 16681-16692.

[25] Muller, M. J. & Baer, H. P. (1983). Relaxant effects of forskolin in smooth muscle. Role of cyclic AMP. *Naunyn-Schmiedeberg's archives of pharmacology,* 322, 78-82.

[26] Lincoln, T. M. & Fisher-Simpson, V. (1984). A comparison of the effects of forskolin and nitroprusside on cyclic nucleotides and relaxation in the rat aorta. *European Journal of Pharmacology,* 101, 17-27.

[27] Kämpfer, N., Lamyel, F., Schütz, I., Warnken, M., Hoffmann, K., von Kügelgen, I. & Racké, K. (2014). Dual regulation of β2-adrenoceptor messenger RNA expression in human lung fibroblasts by β2-cAMP signaling; delayed upregulated inhibitors oppose a rapid in onset, direct

stimulation of gene expression. *Naunyn-Schmiedeberg's archives of pharmacology,* 387, 649-657.

[28] Butler, M. S. (2005). Natural products to drugs: natural product derived compounds in clinical trials. *Natural Product Reports,* 22, 162-195.

[29] Gonzalez-Sanchez, R., Trujillo, X., Trujillo-Hernandez, B., Vásquez, C., Huerta, M., & Elizalde, A. (2006). Forskolin versus sodium cromoglycate for prevention of asthma attacks: a single-blinded clinical trial. *Journal of International Medical Research,* 34, 200-207.

[30] Kotwani, A. (1998) Use of chick embryo in screening for teratogenicity. *Indian Journal of Physiology and Pharmacology,* 42, 189-204.

[31] Hamburger, V. & Hamilton, H. L. (1992). A series of normal stages in the development of the chick embryo. 1951. *Developmental Dynamics,* 195, 231-272.

[32] Metcalfe, J. & Stock, M. K. (1993). Current topic: oxygen exchange in the chorioallantoic membrane, avian homologue of the mammalian placenta. *Placenta,* 14, 605-613.

[33] Ackerman, R. A. & Rahn, H. (1981). In vivo O2 and water vapor permeability of the hen's eggshell during early development. *Respiration Physiology,* 45, 1-8.

[34] Ribatti, D. (2008). Chick embryo chorioallantoic membrane as a useful tool to study angiogenesis. *International Review of Cell and Molecular Biology,* 270, 181-224.

[35] Lindgren, I., Zoer, B., Altimiras, J. & Villamor E. (2010). Reactivity of chicken chorioallantoic arteries, avian homologue of human fetoplacental arteries. *Journal of Physiology and Pharmacology: an official journal of the Polish Physiological Society,* 61, 619-628.

[36] Stewart, R., Nelson, J. & Wilson, D. J. (1990). Growth of the chick area vasculosa *in ovo* and in shell-less culture. *Journal of Anatomy,* 172, 81-87.

[37] Omo-Aghoja L. (2014). Maternal and Fetal Acid-Base Chemistry: A Major Determinant of Perinatal Outcome. *Annals of Medical and Health Sciences Research,* 4, 8-17.

[38] Martisen, B. J. (2005). Reference guide to the stages of chick heart embryology. *Developmental Dynamics*, 233, 1217-1237.

[39] Ignarro, L. J. & Shideman, F. E. (1968). Catechol-O-methyl transferase and monoamine oxidase activities in the heart and liver of the embryonic and developing chick. *Journal of Pharmacology and Experimental Therapeutic,* 159, 29-37.

[40] Lipshultz, S., Shanfeld, J. & Chacko, S. (1981). Emergence of beta-adrenergic sensitivity in the developing chicken heart. *Proceedings of the National Academy of Sciences,* 78, 288-292.

[41] Hejnova, L., Hahnova, K., Kockova, R., Svatunkova, J., Sedmera, D. & Novotny, J. (2014). Adenylyl cyclase signaling in the developing chick heart: the deranging effect of antiarrhythmic drugs. *Biomed Research International,* 2014, 463123.

[42] Smith, C. J. & Pappano, A. J. (1985). A role for adenylate cyclase in the subsensitivity to isoproterenol during ontogenesis of the embryonic chick ventricle. *Journal of Pharmacology and Experimental Therapeutic,* 235, 335-343.

[43] Thakkar, J. K. & Sperelakis, N. (1987). Changes in cyclic nucleotide levels during embryonic development of chick hearts. *Journal of Developmental Physiology,* 9, 497-505.

[44] Hu, C. L., Chandra, R., Ge, H., Pain, J., Yan, L., Babu, G., Depre, C., Iwatsubo, K., Ishikawa, Y., Sadoshima, J., Vatner, S. F. & Vatner, D. E. (2009). Adenylyl cyclase type 5 protein expression during cardiac development and stress. American Journal of Physiology. *Heart and Circulatory Physiology,* 297, H1776-782.

[45] Nishikawa, T., Sato, A., Kanai, T., Kasajima, T., Nakajima, Y., Ando, M. & Takao, A. (1989). The teratogenic effect of forskolin on cardiovascular development in the chick embryo. *Reproductive Toxicology* (Elmsford, N. Y.), 3, 139-142.

[46] Nishikawa, T., Ishiyama, S., Takeda, K. & Kasajima, T. (1995). The effect of forskolin on the teratogenicity of methylxanthines in the chick embryo heart. *Reproductive Toxicology* (Elmsford, N. Y.), 9, 165-168.

[47] Kälin, R. E., Bänziger-Tobler, N. E., Detmar, M. & Brändli, A. W. (2009). An in vivo chemical library screen in Xenopus tadpoles reveals novel pathways involved in angiogenesis and lymphangiogenesis. *Blood,* 114, 1110-1122.

[48] Warren, J. B., Wilson, A. J., Loi, R. K.& Coughlan, M. L. (1993). Opposing roles of cyclic AMP in the vascular control of edema formation. *FASEB Journal: official publication of the Federation of America Societies for Experimental Biology,* 7, 1394-400.

[49] Lindgren, I., Crossley, D. 2nd, Villamor, E. & Altimiras, J. (2011) Hypotension in the chronically hypoxic chicken embryo is related to the β-adrenergic response of chorioallantoic and femoral arteries and not to bradycardia. American Journal of Physiology. *Regulatory, Integrative and Comparative Physiology,* 30, 1161-1168.

In: Forskolin
Editor: Marty H. Walker
ISBN: 978-1-63463-918-7

Chapter 4

FORSKOLIN AND *COLEUS FORSKOHLII*: CLINICAL APPLICATIONS FOR OVERWEIGHT AND OBESITY

Seika Kamohara [1,2,*]
[1]Health Science University, Yamanashi, Japan;
[2]DHC Corporation, Tokyo, Japan

ABSTRACT

Forskolin is a labdane diterpene, isolated from plant *Coleus forskohlii* (Lamiaceae), which has been used in traditional Indian medicine, Ayurveda. Forskolin (7beta-acetoxy-8, 13-epoxy-1a, 6β, 9a-trihydroxy-labd-14-en-11-one) increases the production of cyclic adenosine monophosphatase (cAMP) byactivating adenylate cyclase. Forskolin has many pharmacological effects and some of them are independent of cAMP. *Coleus forskohlii* root, which contains forskolin has been used in Ayurvedic medicine for cardiovascular disorders and gastrointestinal disorders. Recently, forskolin has been used as anti-obesity and anti-glaucoma agents. This chapter aims to summarize pharmacological studies of forskolin towards its clinical applications especially for obesity and metabolic syndrome.

---

* Author's contact address: Seika Kamohara, M.D., Ph.D. Health Science University, Minami-azabu 2-8-12 Nissei-bldg. 11fl. DHC, Tokyo 106-0047, Japan, Phone: +81-3-5442-3945, Fax: +81-3-5442-3947, E-mail: kamohara-seika@umin.ac.jp.

ABBREVIATIONS

BMI	body mass index;
CF	*Coleus forskohlii*;
cAMP	cyclic adenosine monophosphate;
GI	gastrointestinal;
TSH	thyroid stimulating hormone;
T3	triiodothyronine; T4, thyroxine
T4	thyroxine

INTRODUCTION

Coleus forskohlii (Lamiaceae) is an Indian botanical which has been used in Ayurvedic medicine (Figure 1). The root portion contains the active constituent, forskolin. (de Souza, Premila) It is also known originally as coleonol. (Dubey) *Coleus forskohlii*(CF) has been used as a medicinal herb for various kinds of diseases such as hypertension, congestive heart failure, colic, respiratory disorders and asthma. The plant has been cultivated for the use of the root, and commonly consumed as part of an ordinary diet (e.g. pickles, etc.). (de Souza)

In 1974, the diterpene, forskolin, was isolated from the root of CF, which had blood pressure lowering and antispasmodic effects. So far, CF is the only plant source known to have this substance. (Ammon, Jagtap) The various therapeutic effects of forskolin are well-documented as being an anti-platelet,anti-spasmodic, anti-inflammatory, hypotensive, vasodilator, positive inotrophic, smooth muscle relaxant, a bronchodilator, anti-glaucoma agent, and anti-obesity. These are all due to its unique ability to activate the enzyme, adenylate cyclase, in the absence of a functional guanine nucleotide regulatory protein. (Ammon, de Souza)

Forskolin is an adenylate cyclase activator. Adenylate cyclase is involved in the production of cyclic adenosine monophosphate (cAMP), a significant biochemical agent in metabolic processes. (Burns) cAMP induces a reaction of biochemical events that trigger metabolic processes, diet induced thermogenesis, increased lean body mass and stimulate loss of body fat. Therefore, recent use of CF extract is one of the best means to maintain healthy body composition and lean body mass levels. Recently, several trials have reported the anti-obesity effect by the CF extract. (Kamohara, Lieberman)

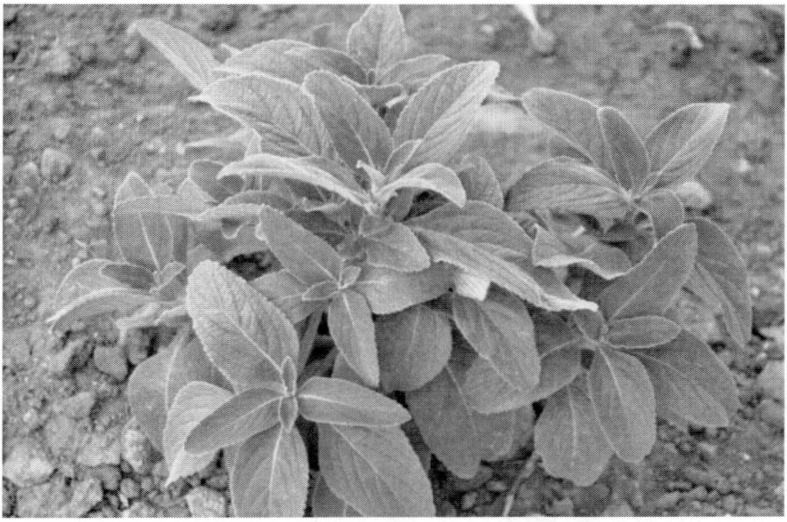

A

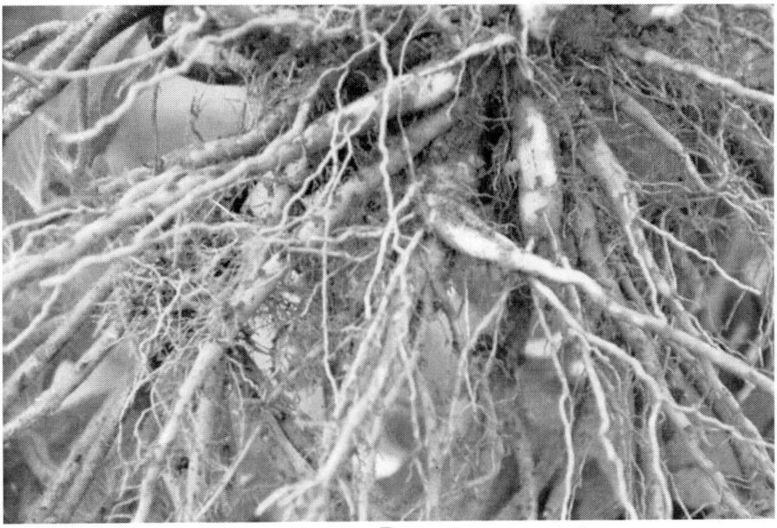

B

Note: A. *Coleus forskohlii* is an Indian herb, which belongs to the family Labiatae. B. Its root has been used in traditional Indian medicine, Ayurveda. All photoscourtesy of DHC Corporation,Tokyo, Japan.

Figure 1. Botanical aspects of *Coleus forskohlii*.

Pharmacology of Forskolin

Sources and Structure

Forskolin is the labdane diterpene, which is found in the root of *Coleus forskohlii.* Its chemical name is 7beta-Acetoxy-8, 13-epoxy-1a, 6β, 9a-trihydroxy-labd-14-en-11-one (Figure 2). (Wagh) Its molecular weight is 410.5 g/mole (anhydrous) and molecular formula is C 22 H 34 O 7.The melting point of forskolin is 228°C-230°C. It is soluble in DMSO, ethanol, methanol and dichloromethane.Its UV absorption maxima are at210 nm and 305 nm. (Wagh)

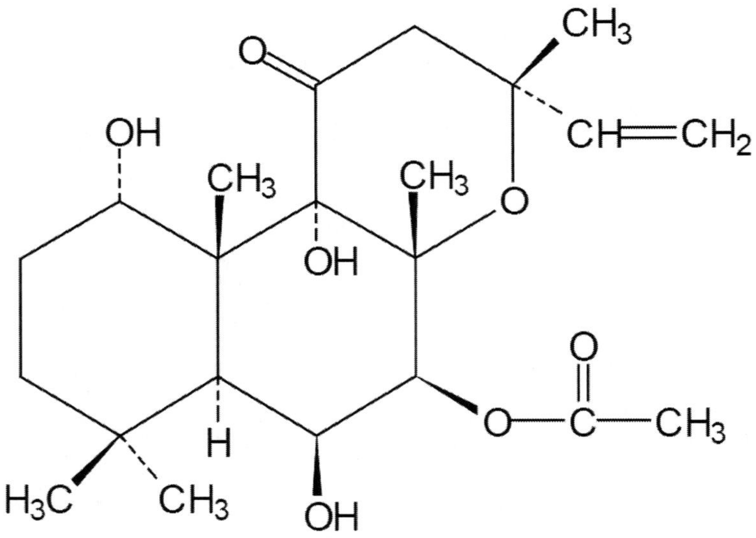

Note:Forskolin is the labdane diterpene, and its molecular formula is C 22 H 34 O 7.

Figure 2. Structure of Forskolin.

Mechanisms of Action

At the Cellular Level

Forskolin activates adenylate cyclase by direct stimulation which leads to the production of cyclic adenosine monophosphatase (cAMP). Many hormones are capable of regulating cAMP, but they do so indirectly. It is unusual for a substance to produce such activation directly.

Activation of adenylate cyclase occurs through a direct action of the diterpene on the catalytic subunit of adenylate cyclase, however, forskolin requires the presence of guanine nucleotide-binding protein, the G8 protein, for maximal stimulation of the enzyme.

Forskolin has been shown to increase cAMP formation in all eukaryotic cells except sperm, without hormonal activation of adenylate cyclase. In vitro studies show that forskolin has many pharmacological effects as follows.

Forskolin and its potentiation of cAMP inhibits platelet aggregation (Agarwal), histamine release from human basophils and mast cells (Marone), and promotes lipolysis induced by forskolin in rat fat cells (Okuda).

Animal Studies

Some of the major pharmacological activities of forskolin are reported in animal studies using *Coleus forskohlii*(CF) extract. For example, forskolin lowers blood pressure in cats and rats (Dubey), lowers intraocular pressure in rabbits (Caprioli), and promotes vasodilation in rabbits (Wysham).

Some of these effects implicate clinical relevance, as detailed below.

In anesthetized rabbits, forskolin (10 micrograms/kg per min) increased blood flow (ml/min per 100 gm) from 39 ± 5 (mean ± S.E.) to 56 ± 9 (p less than 0.05) in cerebrum, and increased flow to myocardium and kidney despite a decrease in mean arterial pressure. Forskolin did not alter cerebral oxygen consumption, which indicated that the increase in cerebral blood flow was a direct vasodilator effect and was not secondary to increased metabolism. (Wysham)

The effects of CFextract on obesity and metabolic syndrome has been shown in animal studies.

In ovariectomized rats, the administration of CF extract reduced body weight, food intake, and fat accumulation (Han). Eight-week-old female Wistar rats were assigned to four groups: a sham-operated group fed the control diet (MF, sham-m) ; an ovx-m group fed the control diet; a sham-operated group fed the control diet containing 50 g/kg of CF extract (sham-c) ; and an ovx-c group fed the control diet containing 50 g/kg ofCF extract. Administration of CF extracts reduced body weight, food intake, and fat accumulation in ovx rats (Han).

Effect of CFextracton cafeteria diet-induced obesity was shownin rat models Shivaprasad. Rats were randomly divided into five groups as follows: normal pellet diet group; cafeteria diet group; cafeteria diet followed by 50 mg/kg/day, 100 mg/kg/dayCF extract, and 45 mg/kg/day orlistat groups, respectively. Obesity was induced by feeding a cafeteria diet in rats. Administration of CF extract significantly halted increase in food intake and weight gain associated with the cafeteria diet. Development of dyslipidemia was also significantly inhibited.

In mice, the possible hepatotoxicity and the induction of hepatic drug metabolizing enzymes by CF extract were reported. (Virgona, Yokotani) Mice were given 0-5% standardized CF extract with 10% forskolin in an AIN 93G-based diet for 3-5 weeks. The CF extract decreased visceral fat weight by between 16% and 63%, and a dose-dependent several folds increase was observed in liver weights and plasma AST (aspartate aminotransferase), ALT (alanine aminotransferase) and ALP (alkaline phosphatase) activities. Liver histology of mice fed 0.5% CF extract for 3 weeks showed hepatocyte hypertrophy and fat deposition. In contrast, none of the hepatic responses measured were altered when mice were given a diet containing pure forskolin alone at the dose corresponding to its content in 0.5% CF extract. This data indicated that forskolin was not involved in the CF extract induced hepatotoxicity and was caused by other unidentified constituents in CFE (Virgona). However, the clinical significance is not clear because there is no hepatotoxicity reported in any human studies.In mice, CF extract might induce hepatic drug metabolizing enzymes, cytochrome P450. However, the mechanism of CYP induction remains unclear.(Yokotani)

CLINICAL STUDIES

Weight Loss and Weight Management

Obesity has become one of the major challenges to public health worldwide. The lack of efficient therapeutics for obesity demands a tailored-made approach. Even though there are currently no effective pharmacological interventions for obesity, the growing body of literature shows the potential efficacy of botanical medicine or phototherapy as a complementary therapy. Several botanicals, including CFhave been used and are considered as an option for treating obesity and weight management.

Overweight and obesity are defined as abnormal or excessive fat accumulation that may impair health. Itis defined in terms of body mass index (BMI), which is calculated as body weight divided by the square of height (kg/m2).The WHO definition is: a BMI greater than or equal to 25 is overweight, and a BMI greater than or equal to 30 is obesity.

The imbalance of energy expenditure and energy intake leads obesity. Daily energy expenditure consists of three components: basal metabolic rate (60–75%), energy expenditure due to physical activity (about 20%) and diet-inducedthermogenesis (about 10%). Thermogenesis is the generation of heat and diet-induced thermogenesis is the energy spent in eating, digesting and assimilating food. Basal metabolism is the minimum amount of energy expended by a conscious person at complete rest. Lean body mass is the mass of the body not including the fat (and also called fat-free mass). Lean body mass is the most important factor influencing resting metabolism.

Forskolin As an Anti-Obesity Agent

Forskolin is an adenylate cyclase activator. Adenylate cyclase is involved in the production of cyclic adenosine monophosphate (cAMP), a significant biochemical agent in metabolic processes. cAMP induces a reaction of biochemical events that trigger metabolic processes, diet induced thermogenesis, increase lean body mass and stimulate loss of body fat. Therefore, recent use of CF extract is a means to maintain healthy body composition and lean body mass levels.

Several trials have reported the anti-obesity effect by forskolin or extract of CF root.

Several clinical trials have reported the weight-loss effect of CF extract. An open-label study of 8 weeks duration reported that 6 overweight, but otherwise healthy, women (BMI > 25) with oral administration of CF extract, containing 50 mg per day of forskolin, resulted in significant reduction of body weight and fat content (Lieberman). In a randomized, double-blind, placebo-controlled 12-week trial, a significant weight loss was observed in 30 overweight/obese men after an intake of CF extract (containing 250 mg per day of 10% forskolin) (Godard). A randomized, double-blind, 12-week clinical trial reported that overweight/obese women (BMI 25–35) taking CF extract (containing 50 mg per day of forskolin) showed weight loss while the placebo group gained weight. Heart rate, blood pressure and blood lipids were unaffected. No clinically significant side effects were observed (Henderson).

Recent Findings from Our Clinical Studies

We conducted an open-label study evaluating the efficacy of the CF root extract for weight management. Fifteen healthy volunteers participated in an 8-weeks open-label study under informed consent. Subjects received 500 mg of CF extracts (10% forskolin), twice a day with meals. Body composition measurements were conducted with the bioelectric impedance analyzer on every week. Body weight (kg), fat content (kg), lean body mass (kg) and basal metabolic rate (kcal) were obtained. Twelve subjects (5 men, 7 women, mean age; 32.0±2.3) completed the study. The significant decreases of BMI(24.92 ± 0.87 to 23.99 ± 0.86, p=0.0038), body weight (66.33±3.00 to 63.96±3.10, p=0.0038), and fat content (29.64±2.19 to 27.77±2.27, p=0.0038) were detected after 8 weeks, compared to the baseline level. Lean body mass (44.34±2.98 to 43.93±3.01, p=0.0044) and basal metabolic rate (1379.1±74.4 to 1363.9±77.5, p=0.0254) were also significantly decreased. (Table 1) Three subjects reported abdominal discomfort, such as increased bowel movements, soft stool and diarrhea. No other clinically significant side effects were found.

Published clinical studies which reported the anti-obesity effect by forskolin or extract of CF root are summarized. (Table 2)

Table 1. Effects of *Coleus forskohlii* extract on body composition

	Baseline	4 weeks	8 weeks	p value
BMI	24.92 ± 0.87	24.26 ± 0.84	23.99 ± 0.86	p = 0.0038
Body weight (kg)	66.33 ± 3.00	64.61 ± 2.99	63.96 ± 3.10	p = 0.0038
Fat content (kg)	29.64 ± 2.19	28.75 ± 2.20	27.77 ± 2.27	p = 0.0038
LBM (kg)	44.34 ± 2.98	44.03 ± 3.02	43.93 ± 3.01	p = 0.0044
BMR (kcal)	1379.1 ± 74.4	1367.6 ± 76.0	1363.9 ± 77.5	p = 0.0254
Systolic BP (mmHg)	116 ± 5	116 ± 5	114 ± 5	p > 0.05 (n.s)
Diastolic BP (mmHg)	73 ± 5	74 ± 5	73 ± 4	p > 0.05 (n.s)

Note: N = 12; BMI, body mass index; LBM, lean body mass; BMR, basal metabolic rate; BP, blood pressure; n.s., not significant.

Values are represented as mean ± standard error.

The p values indicate the difference between values at baseline and at 8 weeks.

Table 2. Evidence list of forskolin or *Coleus forskohlii* extract on obesity and body composition

Representative Reference (Publication year)	Study Design	Subjects (number of subjects)	Daily dose of forskolin or CF extract	Intervention Period	Results
Lieberman SA (2004)	Open-label study	Overweight women (n = 6)	50 mg of forskolin	8 weeks	Significant reduction of body weight and fat content
Godard MP (2005)	Randomized, double-blind, placebo-controlled study	Overweight/obese men (n = 30)	50 mg of forskolin (500 mg of CF extract)	12 weeks	Significant reduction of % body fat and fat mass
Henderson S (2005)	Randomized, double-blind, placebo-controlled study	Overweight/obese women (n = 30)	50 mg of forskolin	12 weeks	Prevented weight gain, while the placebo group gained weight
Kamohara S (2013)	Open-label study	Healthy volunteers (n = 15)	100 mg of forskolin (1,000 mg of CF extract)	8 weeks	Decreased BMI, Fat content, Body weight vs. 0 week

Note: Evidence list of references, study designs, numbers of subjects, intervention periods, and results.

OTHER CLINICAL BENEFITS

Forskolin As Antiglaucoma Molecule

Forskolin has an effect to lower intraocular pressure and it is approved as an antiglaucoma drug in India.The topical application of forskolin is capable of reducing intraocular pressure in rabbits, monkeys, and humans. (Caprioli, Wagh) The study to evaluate effects of forskolinon aqueous humour formation, intraocular pressure and on ciliary epithelial cyclic AMP levels, either in presence or in absence of IBMX, using the bovine isolated arterially perfused eye, excised ciliary processes and cultured ciliary epithelium was conducted. (Shahidullah) Forskolin, which stimulates cyclic AMP synthesis without interacting with cell surface receptors, produced highly significant increases in ciliary cyclic AMP content both in presence and in absence of IBMX, but had no effect on aqueous humour formation in the isolated eye.

In rabbits, net aqueous humor inflow decreases, outflow facility remains unchanged, and ciliary blood flow increases. Tolerance to the intraocular pressure lowering effect did not occur in rabbits after topical doses given every 6 hr for 15 days. In vitro forskolin activates adenylate cyclase of crude particulate homogenates prepared from cultured human ciliary epithelia or from dissected ciliary epithelial processes of rabbit or human eyes. This activation is not blocked by timolol. The stimulation of adenylate cyclase by isoproterenol in vitro is potentiated in the presence of forskolin. (Caprioli) Taken together, forskolin seems to represent a potentially useful class of antiglaucoma agents differing in molecular mechanism of action from previously used drugs.

Treatment of Hypertension

Hypertension, also known as high or raised blood pressure, is a condition in which the blood vessels have persistently raised pressure. Normal blood pressure is defined as a blood pressure of 120 mm Hg when the heart beats (systolic) and a blood pressure of 80 mm Hg when the heart relaxes (diastolic). When systolic blood pressure is equal to or above 140 mm Hg and/or a diastolic blood pressure equal to or above 90 mm Hg the blood pressure is considered as hypertension.

The hypotensive effects of forskolin are observed in deafferented as well as in the spinal transected cat, and suggested that lowering of blood pressure is not mediated by the central effects of forskolin, but is rather due to the direct peripheral vasodilatory actions, through its smooth muscle relaxation property. (Ammon)

In the clinical trial, efficacy of CF extract on hypertension was reported in the middle age and geriatric population. [Jagtap]A total of 49 hypertensive patients were divided in two groups-Group I (CF extract supplementation) and Group II (Churna tablet,a mixture of powdered herbs and or minerals used in Ayurvedic medicine). Out of 27 enrolled patients of group I, 21 patients completed the treatment. In Group II, out of 22 registered patients, a total of

20 patients completed the treatment. On analyzing the overall effect, 76.19% patients in Group I and 75.00% patients in Group II were mildly improved. Comparatively the overall treatment with group I was found to be better. (Jagtap)

Psoriasis

Psoriasis is an autoimmune disease that causes raised, red, scaly patches to appear on the skin. It typically affects the outside of the elbows, knees or scalp, though it can appear on any location. Patients with psoriasis have decreased cAMP and increased GMP in affected areas. Increased cGMP levels are associated with cell proliferation.

The hyporesponsiveness of beta-Adrenergic receptor has been observed in psoriasis and after exposure of epidermis to phorbol esters. Forskolin, which acts synergistically with receptor agonists in elevating endogenous levels of cyclic AMP, is reported a useful probe in defining the mechanism of this decreased responsiveness both in phorbol-ester-treated skin and in psoriasis. (De Vries, Tamura) Theability of forskolin to regulate cAMP levels indermatocytes has been shown to havetherapeutic benefit in alleviation ofpsoriasis.The supplementation of forskolin improved symptoms of psoriasis in patients. (Ammon)

SAFETY OF FORSKOLIN

Findings from Clinical Studies

Forskolin and CF extractappears to be well-tolerated when taken by healthy adults by mouth in suggested doses for up to six months in clinical studies. (Lieberman, Godard, Kamohara, Henderson) There were no major adverse events in any clinical trials. No clinically significant changes were seen in metabolic markers, blood lipids, liver enzymes, electrolytes, hormones (insulin, TSH, T3, and T4), heart rate, and blood pressure. (Kamohara) Minor GI events were reported in the study in Japanese population. (Kamohara)

Cardiovascular Effects

Forskolin or CFextracthas potential hypotensive effect and may lower blood pressure.Forskolin has shown positive inotropic effect on the increase of heart rate and could lower blood pressure in dogs and cats. (Lindner 1978). Coleonol or forskolin lower blood pressure in cats and rats due to relaxation of the vascular smooth muscle. (Dubey) It produced a well-marked and sustained hypotensionin anesthetized cats in the dose range of 0.1 to 1.0mg/kg.It has also been shown that forskolin has a positive inotropic effect on isolated rabbit heart as well as on cat heart in vivo. Forskolin exhibits nonspecific spasmolytic activity on smooth muscle of the gastrointestinal tract in various species but not on bronchial musculature of guinea pigs. (Dubey).

It is important to note that all of these hypotensiveeffects reported within animal models.These effects were not shown in clinical studies to evaluate efficacy and safety of CF on overweight and obesity. (Godard, Kamohara)

In Ayurvedic medicine, it was reported that CF extract supplementation showed mild improvements in the systolic and diastolic blood pressures in geriatric populations with hypertension (Jagtap).

Mechanism of Gastrointestinal Symptoms

The contemporary use of dietary supplements containing CF extract for weight-loss associated with soft stool and diarrhea anecdotally. In our clinical study, three subjects reported mild gastrointestinal adverse events. (Kamohara) Therefore, we performed the dose escalation study of CF supplementation to assess frequency and severity of gastrointestinal (GI) adverse events. Twenty nine healthy subjects were recruited into an open-label trial, and were administered escalating doses from 250 to 1,000 mg for 4-week period. Adverse events were recorded on daily basis. Blood, urine and stool samples were obtained before and after supplementation in a subset of 10 subjects to assess the safety. All 29 subjects completed the study. Intake of CF was associated with minor gastrointestinal adverse events such as soft stool and diarrhea, which appeared to be dose-related. There were no major adverse events. Six or seven subjects reported minor GI events in each dose of CF.

The mechanism of GI events is not fully elucidated, but one possibility is that cAMP induced efflux of Cl-ion from intestinal membrane caused GI events such as soft stool and diarrhea. We suggest the following mechanism as a causality of GI events and CF extract supplementation.

One of processes to establish an osmotic gradient that pulls water into the lumen of the intestine is the activity of crypt cells to secrete electrolytes, leading to water secretion. The lumenal membrane of crypt epithelial cells contains a cyclic AMP-dependent chloride channel known also as the cystic fibrosis transmembrane conductance regulator or CFTR (Thiagarajah). This channel is responsible for secretion of water by the following steps: First, chloride ions enter the crypt epithelial cell by co-transport with sodium and potassium. Then, sodium is pumped back out via sodium pumps, and potassium is exported via a number of channels. Activation of adenylyl cyclase by a number of so-called secretagogues leads to generation of cyclic AMP. Elevated intracellular concentrations of cAMP in crypt cells activate the CFTR, resulting in secretion of chloride ions into the lumen. Accumulation of negatively-charged chloride anions in the crypt creates an electric potential that attracts sodium, pulling it into the lumen, apparently across tight junctions - the net result is secretion of NaCl. Secretion of NaCl into the crypt creates an osmotic gradient across the tight junction and water is drawn into the lumen.

Theoretically, increased level of c-AMP in the intestine led by intake of CF extract could cause secretion of chloride ions into the lumen via the CFTR. This could result in secretion of water, which would be manifested as soft stool and diarrhea. Therefore, forskolin or CF extract could cause GI events by stimulating chloride ion channels.

CONCLUSION

Forskolin from *Coleus forskohlii* extract has various pharmacological activities and it could play a pivotal role to promote well-being and healthy body weight. The supplementation of *Coleus forskohlii* extract may be beneficial for maintaining healthy body composition and lean body mass levels. Further studies are warranted to conclusively demonstrate the effectiveness of forskolin and *Coleus forskohlii* extract for well-being and weight management.

ACKNOWLEDGMENTS

The author is grateful to Dr. L. Todd Landreneau for preparing this manuscript.

REFERENCES

Agarwal KC, Parks RE Jr. Synergistic inhibition of platelet aggregation by forskolin plus PGE1 or 2-fluoroadenosine: Effects of 2, 5-dideoxyadenosine and 5-methylthioadenosine. *Biochem. Pharmacol.* 1982;31:3713-6.

Ammon HP, Müller AB. Forskolin: from an ayurvedic remedy to a modern agent. *Planta Med* 1985;51:473-7.

Burns TW, Langley PE, Terry BE, et al. Comparative effects of forskolin and isoproterenol on the cyclic AMP content of human adipocytes, *Life Sci.* 1987;40: 145-54.

Caprioli J, Sears M, Bausher L. Forskolin lowers intraocular pressure by reducing aqueous inflow. *Invest. Ophthalmol. Vis. Sci.* 1984;25:268-77.

De Vries GW, Amdahl LD, Lowe N, et al.Effect of forskolin on beta-adrenergic hyporesponsiveness in skin. *Skin Pharmacol.* 1988;1:106-14.

de Souza NJ, Dohadwalla AN, Reden J. Forskolin. a labdane diterpenoid with antihypertensive, positive inotropic, platelet aggregation inhibitory, and adenylate cyclase activating properties. *Med. Res .Rev.* 1983;3:201-19.

Dubey MP, Srimal RC, Nityanand S, Dhawan BN. Pharmacological studies on coleonol, a hypotensive diterpene from Coleus forskohlii. *J. Ethnopharmacol.* 1981;3:1-13.

Godard MP, Johnson BA, Richmond SR. Body composition and hormonal adaptations associated with forskolin consumption in overweight and obese men. *Obesity Research* 2005;13:1335-43.

Han LK, Morimoto C, Yu RH, et al. Effects of Coleus forskohlii on fat storage in ovariectomized rats. *Yakugaku Zasshi* 2005;125:449-53.

Henderson S, Magu B, Rasmussen C, et al. Effects of Coleus forskohlii supplementation on body composition and hematological profiles in mildly overweight women. *J. Int. Soc. Sports Nutr.* 2005;2:54-62.

Jagtap M, Chandola HM, Ravishankar B. Clinical efficacy of Coleus forskohlii (Willd.) Briq. (Makandi) in hypertension of geriatric population. *Ayu* 2011;32:59-65.

Kamohara S and Noparatanawong S. Safety and efficacy of a Coleus forskohlii formulation in healthy volunteers. *Personalized Medicine Universe*. 2013; 2:25–27.

Lichey I, Friedrich T, Priesnitz M, Biamino G, Usinger P, Huckauf H. Effect of forskolin on methacholine-induced bronchoconstriction in extrinsic asthmatics. *Lancet* 1984;2:167.

Lieberman SA. A new potential weapon for fighting obesity. forskolin—the active diterpene in Coleus. *Alternative Complementary Therapy* 2004;10:330-3.

Lindner E, Dohadwalla AN, Bhattacharya BK.Positive inotropic and blood pressure lowering activity of a diterpene derivative isolated from Coleus forskohli: Forskolin. *Arzneimittelforschung*. 1978;28:284-9.

Marone G, Columbo M, Triggiani M, Vigorita S, Formisano S. Forskolin inhibits the release of histamine from human basophils and mast cells. *Agents Actions*. 1986 Apr;18(1-2):96-9.

Metzger H, Lindner E. The positive inotropic-acting forskolin, a potent adenylate cyclase activator. Arzneimittelforschung 1981;31:1248-50.

Okuda H, Morimoto C, Tsujita T. Relationship between cyclic AMP production and lipolysis induced by forskolin in rat fat cells. *J. Lipid Res.* 1992;33:225-31.

Premila MS. Ayurvedic Herbs: A Clinical Guide to the Healing Plants of Traditional Indian Medicine, Routledge, New York, 2006.

Shivaprasad HN, Gopalakrishna S, Mariyanna B, et al.Effect of Coleus forskohlii extract on cafeteria diet-induced obesity in rats. *Pharmacognosy Res.* 2014;6:42-5.

Tamura T, Takahashi H, Ishida-Yamamoto A, et al. Functional alteration of guanine nucleotide binding proteins (Gs and Gi) in psoriatic epidermis. *J. Dermatol. Sci*. 1998;17:61-6.

Thiagarajah JR, Verkman AS. CFTR pharmacology and its role in intestinal fluid secretion. *Curr. Opin. Pharmacol.* 2003;3:594-9.

Virgona N, Taki Y, Yamada S, et al. Dietary Coleus forskohlii extract generates dose-related hepatotoxicity in mice. *J. Appl. Toxicol.* 2013;33:924-32.

Wagh VD, Dehghan MH, Wagh KV, Salve SA, Tandale YN. Pharmacological potential and phytopharmaceutics of Coleus forskohlii (Makandi): A review. *J. GMP Ind. Pharm.* 2009;3:50-4.

Wagh VD, Patil PN, Surana SJ, Wagh KV.Forskolin: upcoming antiglaucoma molecule. *J. Postgrad. Med.* 2012;58:199-202.

Wysham DG, Brotherton AF, Heistad DD. Effects of forskolin on cerebral blood flow: Implications for a role of adenylate cyclase. *Stroke* 1986;17:1299-03.

Yokotani K, Chiba T, Sato Y, et al.Influence of dietary macronutrients on induction of hepatic drug metabolizing enzymes by Coleus forskohlii extract in mice. *J. Nutr. Sci. Vitaminol*. 2013;59:37-44.

INDEX

B

C

D

E

F

G

H

I

J

K

L

M

N

O

P

R

S

T